HOW TO BE A
MINDFUL
DRINKER

HOW TO BE A
MINDFUL
DRINKER

Cut down, take a break, or quit

 Dru Jaeger, Anja Madhvani, Laura Willoughby, Jussi Tolvi and the Club Soda community

CONTENTS

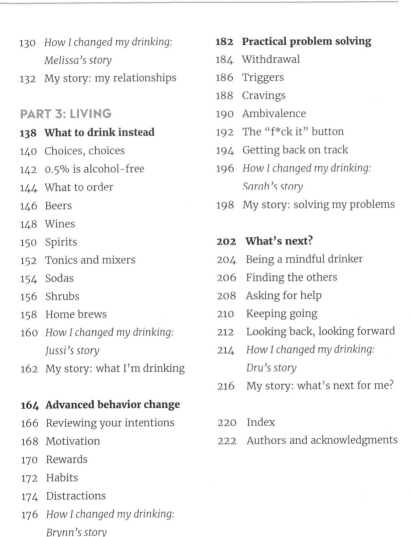

WELCOME TO CLUB SODA

We all have different reasons for wanting to change our drinking. Maybe we've had one hangover too many. Maybe we want better ways to unwind at the end of a stressful day. Maybe we stopped for a month and we want to keep going. Maybe we worry that we wouldn't be sociable without a drink in our hands. Or maybe we know, deep down, that we're drinking more than we want to.

Whatever your reasons for wanting to change your drinking, you're welcome in Club Soda.

Club Soda was born out of our founder Laura's experience of changing her drinking back in 2012. You can read more about her story later in this book (see page 36). Having changed her drinking, she wanted to help other people, too. And so a group of us got together to start Club Soda.

At first, we only wanted to help people change their drinking. We knew that drinking was a social activity for lots of people, but we learned that too many people were struggling to change on their own, and cutting themselves off from others. So, we worked out how changing your drinking could also be a social activity, just like drinking had been, and we built a thriving online and real-world community to make that possible.

We realized people wanted better choices when they went out, so we started running social events and launched a venue guide for mindful drinkers. We started working with the drinks industry, promoting choice in no- and low-alcohol drinks, and so our mindful drinking festivals were born. We discovered we were building a mindful drinking movement. We want to create a world where nobody feels out of place if they're not drinking alcohol.

In Club Soda, we'll never tell you what you should drink or how you should change. You are the best judge of what works for you.

In this book, we'll invite you to try things out, ask you questions to help you reflect, and help you develop new skills. You'll hear stories from people who have changed their drinking. And you'll discover tips from Club Soda members.

It's up to you to decide what you want to drink, in ways that work for you. We'll support you, whatever you decide.

Joining Club Soda makes you part of this mindful drinking movement. You're not just changing your drinking, you're changing the world, too.

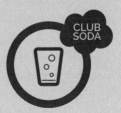

Dru, Anja, Laura, Jussi, and the Club Soda community
joinclubsoda.com

ABOUT MINDFUL DRINKING

Let's start with a question: what is mindful drinking? Mindfulness is everywhere, but it's more than meditation. In its essence, mindfulness is about increasing awareness of ourselves and the world around us. As we learn to pay attention, we can begin to live with intention. Learning both these skills might be one of the keys to our long-term well-being.

But drinking and mindfulness seem to pull in opposite directions. You could argue it's impossible to be mindful and drunk, and you'd have a point. So does the idea of mindful drinking even make sense? We think it does, and we'll explain why.

PAYING ATTENTION

Being a mindful drinker is about increasing awareness of the effect that alcohol has on us, and recognizing how we use it to relate to the world around us. As mindful drinkers, we pay attention to how we feel after one drink, rather than mindlessly plowing on to the next. We notice the effects of alcohol on our physical and our mental well-being. We pay attention to how we react in social situations.

Paying attention roots us firmly in the present, the here and now. What matters most is what is happening in this very moment. Once we have started to pay attention, we can begin to change.

LIVING WITH INTENTION

The other essential part of mindful drinking is acting and living with intention. An intention, if it's a term you've not yet met, is a mindful state where we commit ourselves to actions—what we want and plan to do.

Thinking about the changes we'd like to make helps us discover the life that we imagine and the role that we want alcohol to play in it. We come to

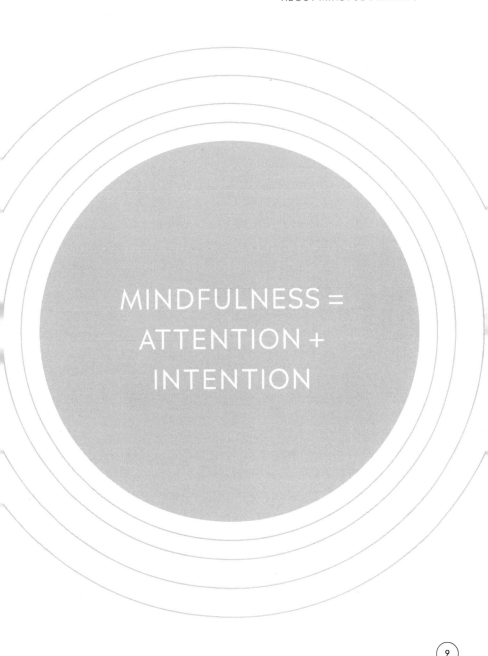

MINDFULNESS =
ATTENTION +
INTENTION

appreciate our limits. We learn to make solid plans that address where, when, what, who with, and how much we want to drink. We begin to see the obstacles in our way as a gift that can help us learn more about ourselves and the world. We grow in confidence relating to the world just as we are, without the need for a drink in our hands.

Living with intention, much like paying attention, focuses us on the here and now, today. Because right now is the only moment we have to change our lives for the better. Becoming a mindful drinker will help you to pay attention and to live with intention.

And this book will show you how to do both.

ABOUT CHANGING YOUR DRINKING

Mindful drinking is for everyone, not just those of us who run into deep difficulties with alcohol.

Alcoholic is a word we avoid using, and you won't hear it often, if at all, from Club Soda members. It's important to know that the scientific evidence on alcoholism is contested, particularly the idea that it is an incurable illness.

Alcoholism is an old-fashioned shorthand for a bundle of issues that might include physical, psychological, and social dependency; compulsive behavior; habitual patterns; and emotional challenges. Seeing all those elements as one thing, rather than their individual parts, makes them appear so complex it's difficult to know where to start untangling them. It's hardly surprising, then, that people take an "all or nothing" approach in response.

But there's an even deeper problem with the concept of alcoholism. When we describe some people as alcoholics, we make them different from the rest of us. We might drink a lot, but at least we're not alcoholics, right? We can use the idea of alcoholism as a way of comforting ourselves that our drinking is OK because it's not as bad as someone else's.

But we're comparing ourselves with the wrong group. We've ignored the fact that most people don't drink heavily and don't drink every day. What's more, we've failed to notice how drinking makes us feel.

In Club Soda, you'll meet members who change their drinking by quitting. Some of them try moderating first. Others take a break and discover it's so good they don't want to start again. What they share in common is a conviction that being "alcohol-free" works for them.

But you'll also meet lots of members who moderate their drinking. They might stop for a bit, cut down by having regular non-drinking days, limit the number of drinks they have on a night out, swap to lower-alcohol alternatives, never drink at home, or go for long stretches of not drinking at all but enjoy a glass of wine on their birthday or other special occasions. There are seemingly endless ways to moderate your drinking, as you become clear about the part you want alcohol to play in your life.

There's no right or wrong way to change your drinking. This book will help you discover the role you want alcohol to play in your life. You'll come to a conclusion for yourself about whether quitting or moderating will work for you. And it's OK to reassess what works for you, make new plans, and try new approaches.

But we also hope this book will help you realize that drinking—and changing your drinking—isn't the most important thing.

What matters is living the life you imagine.

What matters is "becoming who you are," and we'll talk more about what this means on the next page.

ABOUT CHANGING YOUR LIFE

In Club Soda, we talk about **"becoming who you are."**

It's a curious idea, and one that may be easier to experience than to explain. But we should describe what we mean when we say it, and what we think it means about how people change.

If we are drinking more than we want to, for much longer than we want to, and particularly if we have tried to change our drinking before, we can end up not liking ourselves very much.

It's a hard thing to admit that, honestly, we'd rather not be ourselves. We'd rather not have our history, our worries, and the challenges of our day-to-day lives. Some of us drink more than we want to because it makes dealing with those things easier, albeit temporarily.

Whether we're drinking at home alone, with our partner, with friends, or with work colleagues, alcohol can become so woven into the fabric of our lives that we begin to wonder if life would be the same without it.

HOW WE CHANGE

When we change our drinking, our lives begin to change, too. **Two things happen:**

- **First, we begin to reclaim the time and energy that drinking has taken from us.** We begin to completely inhabit the unique place in the world that only we can occupy. We start to live all the way up to the surface of our skin and stop hiding away inside ourselves.
- **Second, we begin to accept those things about ourselves that we don't like.** We find new ways of dealing with them. We begin to see the challenges and difficulties as gifts, not just because they help us grow, but because they are an essential part of the person we are. We wear our scars with pride.

It's these two threads of change together that mean we become who we are. We're not transformed into different people but we don't stay stuck either. Our lives change, but not so much that we stop recognizing ourselves. As we change what we can and accept what we can't, we become who we were always meant to be.

So, that's what we mean by becoming who we are. As we said, it might be easier to experience than to explain.

ABOUT THIS BOOK

It's worth saying up-front what you won't find in the pages of this book. You may have gathered that we're not going to tell you to quit drinking. In fact, we're not going to tell you to do anything. We don't need you to admit that you are powerless over alcohol. We won't challenge you to be sober for the next 12 months as some kind of macho test. Everything in this book is an invitation to explore, to experiment, and to decide for yourself.

We won't give you lots of information about how drinking may be damaging your health. We suspect you know this already. You probably also know all about the low-risk drinking limits. If they had any effect, you would have stopped or cut down already, so you won't find them here either.

This book isn't a substitute for medical advice. If you are physically dependent on alcohol—for example, needing a drink in the morning to feel normal or feeling ill and experiencing shakes when you stop—please talk to a medical professional alongside reading this book. If you're a dependent drinker, it's important not to stop drinking suddenly. The section on withdrawal (see page 184) will help you understand why.

Finally, we're not going to try to convince you to change your drinking. Even if someone gave you this book because they are worried about you, please put it down right now. Come back when you're ready. We mean it. People join Club Soda because they know that they want to change their drinking. We just help them figure out how.

And that's where this book comes in. It's the ultimate how-to guide to becoming a mindful drinker. In it, you'll discover the best of everything we know about how to change your drinking.

- **Part 1: Beginning** starts where you are now, by helping you pay attention to your drinking and how you feel about it. You'll also explore the part you want alcohol to play in your life, and discover some basic tools that will get you started. So expect lots of questions and a fair amount of soul searching, but with plenty of pointers along the way. Time spent now preparing yourself for your mindful drinking journey is time well spent. By the end of Part 1 you'll be armed and ready for what comes next.

- **Part 2: Changing** explores what to expect as you begin to change your drinking. When you are drinking mindfully and noticing all aspects of your drinking, you'll be able to see just how alcohol affects various parts of your life—the effects on your physical well-being, your emotional life, and your relationships with other people—but we'll break it down for you, too.

- **Part 3: Living** explores what it means to live as a mindful drinker. You'll find tips on what to drink if you're not drinking—from no- and low-alcohol beers, wines, and spirits to shrubs, tonics, and home brews—an advanced-behavior change toolkit (which builds on those in Part 1), and practical problem-solving advice for any challenges you face, as well as some thoughts on keeping going for the long term.

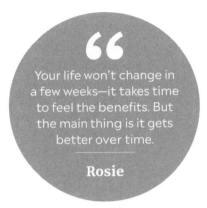

> **"**
>
> Your life won't change in a few weeks—it takes time to feel the benefits. But the main thing is it gets better over time.
>
> **Rosie**

MAKING THE MOST OF THIS BOOK

You could read this book cover to cover, but our experience is that the journey of changing your drinking isn't a linear path with a clear starting point, a defined ending, and a straight line in between; it's more like a winding trail.

So, rather than thinking of this book as a route map to follow slavishly, consider it a map of a landscape that you are beginning to explore for the first time. You will find some signposts along the way (see overleaf for starters). Much of what you will discover applies whether you are quitting or moderating. But if there are significant differences, we'll point them out.

Like any explorer, take notes so you remember where you've been. To help get you started, at the end of every chapter you'll find a handful of note pages that reflect on some of the ideas and suggestions that we've just covered. You can fill in these pages or, if you prefer, copy them out into your own notebook— whatever works best for you. Taking notes can help you retrace your steps if you get lost. And as with any journey, you start where you are.

NOT SURE WHERE TO BEGIN?

Uncertain whether drinking is a problem for you?

Not sure if you can change your drinking?

Ready to make a start?

Taking a month off drinking?

Curious about what to drink instead?

Tried to change your drinking before?

• • • • Dive into the section on becoming mindful and see what you learn about yourself **(see page 24)**.

• • • • Go straight to the inspirational stories of Club Soda members who are featured in this book, like Laura's **(see page 36)**.

• • • • The second chapter is full of useful advice on clarifying intentions, making plans, and tracking your progress **(see page 46)**.

• • • • Part 2 will help you understand some of the immediate effects of changing your drinking on your health, your mood, and your social life **(see page 72)**.

• • • • Start with the guide to choosing the best no- and low-alcohol drinks in Part 3 **(see page 136)**.

• • • • Our advanced behavior-change toolkit and problem-solving guide might be just what you need **(see page 164)**.

If you need advice or encouragement, or you just want to tell someone about what's going on, remember you're not alone. Head straight to the section on finding the others (see page 206) and join us online (joinclubsoda.com).

This first part of the book—as you might expect—is about how to begin. As you work your way through its pages, you will learn the basics of what it is to become a mindful drinker.

Mindful drinking is as simple as paying attention and living with intention. So, first, we'll show you how to pay attention to your drinking and to the reasons why you want to change. Next, we'll help you explore your intentions for the life you want to live. Then, as you begin to find out how you want drinking to fit into your life, we'll guide you to make plans that don't rely on willpower alone. By the end of the second chapter, you'll feel more yourself and you'll be ready to step seamlessly into the next phase of this adventure.

You're setting out on a journey toward becoming who you are. Good things lie ahead. And we're at your side, every step of the way.

Are you ready? Then let's begin.

PART 1

BEGINNING

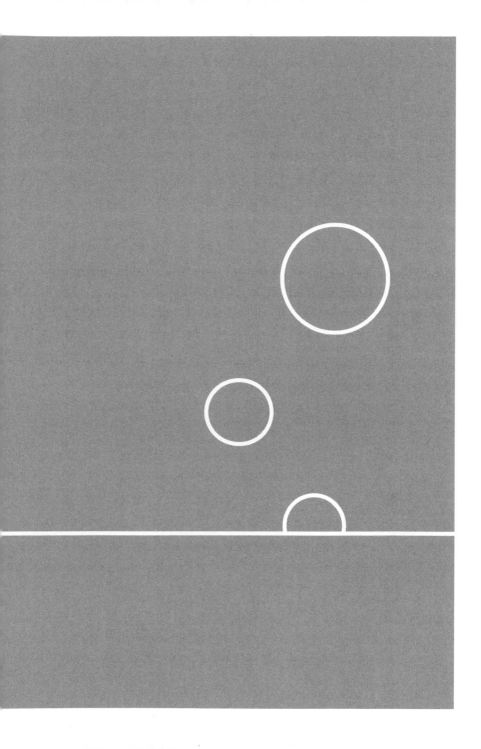

YOU AND YOUR DRINKING

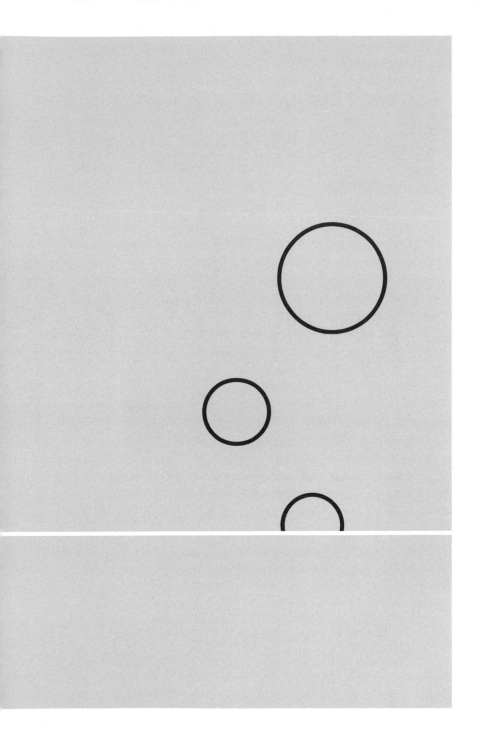

STARTING WHERE YOU ARE

Alcohol can affect our moods, our perceptions, and our relationships (see pages 90–107 and 110–133). But it's not magic. It doesn't change us into different people. You might not believe it right now, but as you change your drinking, you may learn some surprising things about yourself:

If you drink to feel more confident in social situations, the confidence comes from you, not the alcohol.

If drinking helps you relax at the end of the day, the feelings of calm are yours, not alcohol's.

If alcohol cheers you up, you are drawing on the happiness that is already in you, not in a bottle.

You will discover that this is also true of less positive things. If you are drinking to deal with problems in your life, changing your drinking isn't going to make those difficulties disappear. They are still going to be there and you will find new ways to deal with them. Yes, you can change your drinking. And, yes, you are still going to be you.

LIFE IN TECHNICOLOR

Some Club Soda members say that the experience of changing their drinking is like living life in high definition: everything becomes brighter, stronger, and clearer. It's not that you turn into a different person. It feels like you become a more "you" version of you.

The paradox of change is that it happens when we become who we are, not when we try to become what we are not. Positive change is about letting go of old ways of being. Like clearing a flower bed that's overgrown with weeds, it creates space for us to flourish.

You can put a lot of energy into imagining a new life for yourself. But if you're not careful, this new life will be a fantasy, because it won't include you. The only thing anyone can say for certain about their future is that they are going to be part of it.

CHOOSE YOUR ATTITUDES

As you journey toward your future, there are a few attitudes that are useful. Every day:

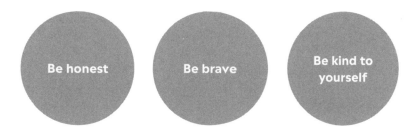

Be honest **Be brave** **Be kind to yourself**

You'll find adopting these attitudes gets easier with daily practice. Together, they will foster a deepening sense of self-acceptance—that means learning to accept yourself with all your strengths and positive attributes as well as all your faults and failings. You'll learn to accept your imperfections, your cracks, and your blemishes. You'll also find ways to accept even those things about yourself that you actively dislike.

This is an ongoing process, maybe even a lifetime's work. But for now, remember this: change is about becoming who you are.

BECOMING MINDFUL

If you've been drinking more than you want to for any length of time, and if you've tried and failed to change your drinking before, you have probably asked yourself "why?": Why do I drink too much?, Why can't I stop when I want to?, and Why am I struggling to change?

"Why?" sounds like a helpful question. When you use it well, it can help you discover things about yourself that you haven't noticed before. But depending on your frame of mind, dwelling on "why?" can easily turn into asking "why me?" As you sink into self-pity, you can imagine that there is something fundamentally wrong with you and start blaming yourself.

As a mindful drinker, you'll learn not to beat yourself up with the question "why?" Mindfulness is about paying attention and that requires different questions that help you notice:

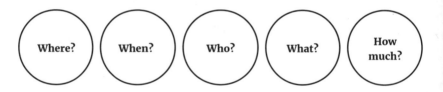

Ask yourself these questions (see pages 38–41). When you answer, be honest and brave. Be kind to yourself, too—remember not to judge yourself or anyone else harshly. All you are doing at this stage is noticing (see box, opposite). Your answers will help you with the practicalities of changing your drinking. Take notes to capture any insights that emerge or anything else that strikes you.

WHERE?

Begin by noticing where you drink. Your environment has a profound impact on your behavior. For example, when you are home alone is there anything

LEARNING HOW TO NOTICE

One of the simplest but most useful mindfulness techniques is to notice things. Let's use an example to help you understand.

Imagine seeing a bird fly above your head. You might be curious about where the bird is going, remark on the color of its wings, or even think that it is beautiful. But it's unlikely that you would get emotionally wrapped up in the experience. You wouldn't judge the bird for how well it flies and you certainly wouldn't obsess about it when it's out of sight.

Mindfulness takes this same approach but applies it to what's going on inside and around us. A thought or feeling is just like the bird in the sky. We can simply and calmly notice it, and then watch it as it flies away.

Noticing can take practice. So start by naming things as they are, but don't dwell on them. As you notice a feeling, say to yourself: "I feel this right now, and it's just a feeling. I can acknowledge it and then let it go."

to stop you opening another bottle? Drinking in a bar or restaurant, or another public space, can feel altogether different from the private world at home, and not just because other people are serving drinks. For instance, you have to ask yourself how you will get home. Or maybe that's a bit of your night that you don't remember.

It may be that drinking is a problem for you everywhere, but it's more likely that there are specific locations where you drink more than you want to. Thinking back over the last month, ask yourself the following:

- **Where** did I drink alcohol?
- **Where** did I not drink alcohol (if I had the opportunity)?
- **Where** was I when I had more to drink than I wanted to?

WHEN?

Next, notice when you drink. You might drink at particular times of day or on specific days of the week. You might notice regular sequences of events—drinks after work or wine with an evening meal—or one-off occasions. The time you put into drinking might well surprise you, but remember not to judge yourself. Thinking back over the last month, ask yourself the following:

• **When** did I drink alcohol?
• **When** did I not drink alcohol (if I had the opportunity)?
• **When** did I drink more than I wanted to?

WHO?

Who you drink with is an important question if alcohol is a big part of your social life. But even if you drink in secret, it's important to consider who you might be hiding your drinking from. When asking who you drink with—or who you avoid when you are drinking—remember to be nonjudgmental; this isn't an exercise in blaming others or yourself. Thinking back over the last month, ask yourself the following:

• **Who** did I drink with?
• **Who** did I not drink with (if I had the opportunity)?
• **Who** was I with when I drank more than I wanted to?

WHAT?

It is a rare person who will drink absolutely anything. Noticing what you drink is about paying attention to your preferences and choices.

People drink beer, wine, and spirits in different contexts, at different paces, and with different people. Paying attention to what you drink gives you more information to deepen your understanding about where and when you are drinking, as well as who you drink with. Thinking back over the last month, ask yourself the following:

- **What** did I drink?
- **What** did I not drink (if I had the opportunity)?
- **What** did I drink when I drank more than I wanted to?

HOW MUCH?

Answering this question is a little different from the previous ones. Rather than reviewing the last month, instead start paying attention now and over the next week to how much you are drinking. You don't need to calculate standard drinks; you only need to be able to count in everyday terms: a glass of wine, a gin and tonic, a pint of beer. That said, even this is trickier than you might think. One reason being that after a certain number of drinks, you may begin to lose count. Another reason is that the act of counting might lead you to change your drinking. Try to approach this exercise with a spirit of curiosity so you can notice your behavior exactly as it is.

One idea is to keep count visually. Over the next seven days take a photo with your phone of every single drink (alcoholic and nonalcoholic). It doesn't matter what it is. Just press the camera button to capture it every time. Inevitably you will forget some drinks. But as you build this visual record, it will reveal exactly how much you are drinking.

PUTTING IT ALL TOGETHER

Take time to review everything.
- What surprises you?
- How do you feel about what you have noticed?
- What clues does this information give you about how you might change your drinking (see pages 52–53)?

> 66
> I thought about the impact of drinking, noticing that I'd feel down the next day or that I'd spend more money on things like takeout.
>
> **Laura**

STORIES ABOUT DRINKING

Our lives are unfolding stories that we tell ourselves. Those stories have good times and bad times. They are full of twists and turns, shock surprises, and exciting revelations. There are many unfinished threads. There are long periods of time in which not much happens at all. And for many of us, alcohol has been a part of the story for as long as we can remember.

As we start to look at stories about drinking, it's key to remember that we're not searching for remnants of some childhood trauma or for some deep-seated reasons behind our drinking. This isn't therapy. Instead, what's important now is to discover the stories you tell yourself about your drinking.

YOUR FIRST DRINK

What is the first drink you remember? Cast your mind back:
- What was going on in your life?
- Was it a good time or a bad time?
- How did the drink make you feel?
- What did that experience reveal about you and drinking?

From that first drink, every drink has taught you something new or reinforced a story you believe about yourself and the world. But it's important to know that all those stories can be rewritten.

REWRITING THE STORY

One way to creatively rewrite your stories is through a process that's known as storyboarding. On a blank piece of paper or in a notebook, draw out eight boxes, or use the ready-made version included on pages 42–43.

In each of the first seven boxes, capture a moment in your life that involved alcohol, starting with the first drinking experience you've just recalled. Capture the good times, the bad times, and significant life moments.

You'll know what really stands out for you.

Common themes do emerge in such stories about, for instance, celebrating with drink, drinking to cope with work, realizing the bottle recycling is growing each week, and wanting to make a new start for your family. But your moments are your own, so it's important to be honest about these to get the most out of this storyboarding exercise.

As you sketch each experience in its box, notice particularly what it told you about you and drinking. Write a short phrase to capture that.

Now, take a moment to look back over the first seven boxes. Do you notice any patterns? Any common threads? What are the stories about drinking that emerge? The final box is a glimpse of your future. What's going to happen next in your story? What do you imagine this to be?

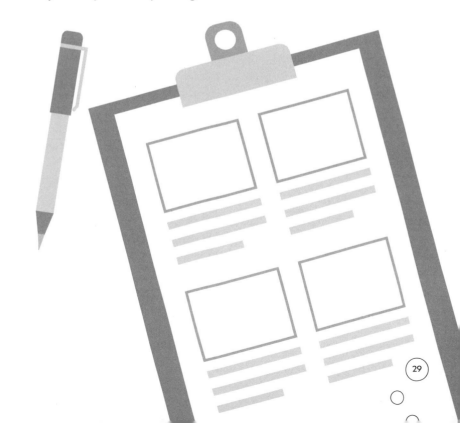

STORIES WE TELL OURSELVES

As you look over your storyboard, you'll have noticed the stories you have told yourself about drinking in the past. Some of those stories are not true now and some of them could hold you back. It's time to let those stories go.

We asked Club Soda members about the stories they needed to let go of as they began to change their drinking. Shown opposite are some of the stories they stopped believing. Read all the way down the list. Any of those sound familiar? Thinking about these stories and your own, what stories about drinking are getting in the way of the life you imagine?

And it might not just be stories you need to let go of. Are there roles you inhabit that don't fit you anymore? Are you, for instance, the one your friends rely on to share a bottle of wine in tough times? What's holding you back from the life you imagine? What are you willing to let go of to become who you are?

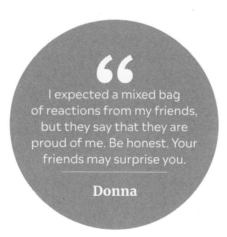

66

I expected a mixed bag of reactions from my friends, but they say that they are proud of me. Be honest. Your friends may surprise you.

Donna

Stories Club Soda members stopped believing

Everyone drinks.

I like the taste of alcohol.

I only drink the good stuff.

Life is no fun without drinking.

A certain amount of alcohol is good for you.

Champagne makes a wedding special.

I will be missing out if I don't drink.

I need alcohol to relax.

Drinking will make me feel better.

I deserve a drink.

I can't imagine life without alcohol.

I am too busy to give up.

I won't fit in if I give up.

I am a hopeless case.

I just don't have any willpower.

I'll have to avoid seeing my friends.

Having an alcohol-free beer is cheating.

I have a disease that can't be cured.

I can't stop because the cravings are too bad.

I won't get promoted if I don't drink with my colleagues.

WILLPOWER HAS ITS LIMITS

We all face the same dilemma. There are things in our lives that give us intense pleasure in the short-term, but the same things can cause us pain in the long-term. Think about, for instance: risky behavior, impulse spending, junk food, and alcohol.

How can we possibly choose between pleasure that is real right now, and pain that might come in the future? When you consider how unbalanced that choice is, it is a wonder that anyone ever exerts willpower at all? And yet we try.

EXHAUSTING WILLPOWER

One way of imagining willpower is as a store of energy that can be used up. We can recharge it, which is why a good night's sleep gives us a chance to start again. But we run the risk of exhausting it each day.

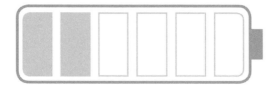

The depletion of willpower reminds us of two things:
- changing through willpower alone is hard work
- trying to change too many things at once can reduce our chances of success.

One way we can avoid relying on willpower alone is by making good decisions easier and bad decisions harder.

DON'T BLAME YOURSELF

Now you know how difficult it is to make good decisions, you can stop blaming yourself that things haven't worked out before.

This probably isn't the first time you've decided to change your drinking. Maybe you took a month off drinking, but found it tricky to keep up with the social events without a glass of alcohol in hand; then, before you knew it, you had simply returned to drinking in the same mode as before. Maybe you tried to cut down, but the amount you drank slowly crept up again. It's easily done.

It's not just you. Willpower tells us that we are missing out on a good thing, so relying on willpower leaves us craving even more. Willpower does have a part to play—it's good in a crisis, for instance—but we need to acquire certain other skills, too.

MAKING GOOD DECISIONS EASIER

Decision-making skills can be learned. Making good decisions easier and bad decisions harder comes down to:

- being clear about your intentions and how you want to change your drinking.
- having practical plans that address all the questions around your drinking (where, when, who with, what, and how much).
- understanding how you'll keep track of your progress, to help you pay attention to things that are going well or not.

The next chapter will help you develop these skills (see page 46). Such skills are a useful addition to the attitudes you are already practicing—being honest, being brave, and being kind to yourself—and everything you've learned so far through paying attention.

We all change our drinking in different ways, but we all share one thing in common: we don't rely on willpower alone.

DISCOVERING YOUR "WHY?"

We're only at the end of the first chapter but you've come so far. Let's review.

- You're practicing being honest, being brave, and being kind to yourself.
- You've become mindful about where, when, who with, what, and how much you drink.
- You've explored the stories you tell yourself about drinking and let some go.
- You've peeked into your future.
- You've discovered you need more than willpower.
- You've learned that changing your drinking is about becoming who you are.

THE DECISION BALANCE SHEET

Remember how you used the question "why?" to beat yourself up? Well, now it's time to put it to good use—to explore the reasons why you want to change your drinking.

When weighing a decision, it helps to look beyond the obvious pros and cons. A tool we like to use to do this is the decision balance sheet. As well as considering the upsides and downsides of changing, the decision balance sheet also prompts you to consider the possibility of not changing. You can see an example of a decision balance sheet on drinking on the opposite page; find a blank one to complete yourself on pages 44–45.

Take time to reflect on everything you've learned so far about yourself and your drinking. Then identify and write in your thoughts on the upsides and the downsides in each of the four boxes.

Give each item in each box a score out of 10, depending on how much it matters to you (10 being most important; 1 being least important). Then add up the scores for each of the boxes. Hopefully, you'll see that the reasons why you want to change your drinking (boxes B and C) outweigh the reasons why not (boxes A and D).

Weighing decisions about drinking

A DECISION BALANCE SHEET	UPSIDES (what will be good, benefits, gains)		DOWNSIDES (what will be difficult, risks, losses)	
Staying the same (not changing drinking)	Stick to routines	3	Letting myself down	10
	After-work drinks	5	Health only going to get worse?	7
	Nothing else ...?	0		
	A =	8	**B =**	17
Changing drinking	Feel happier about myself	9	Unsure how friends will react	2
	Hangover-free family time	10	Tricky conversations with partner	7
	Lose weight?	6	Life might not be as fun?	4
	Feel in control	8		
	C =	33	**D =**	13

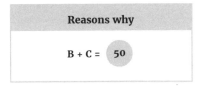

Reasons why	Reasons why not
B + C = **50**	A + D = **21**

LAURA IS THE FOUNDER OF CLUB SODA
AND GAVE UP DRINKING IN 2012

HOW I CHANGED MY DRINKING: **LAURA'S STORY**

Like most of my peers, I started drinking at 14. We were part of the ladette generation and, for us, equality meant being seen pint in hand. Fast forward to university and it was amazing how quickly I could drink two bottles of wine.

I worked in politics and was always ready for a post-meeting drink. I have fond memories of times in the pub, but looking back I see that I was continually inching toward more. I also knew I was my father's daughter when it came to drinking and that worried me, even more so when alcohol contributed to his early death when I was 30. He was only 56. But a job I hated had created the perfect conditions for an already heavy drinking habit to mutate into something self-destructive. I worried about where it could lead if I carried on.

By my mid-thirties, my ability to be able to say "I've had enough" had completely vanished. People would leave the pub, and I'd go to the liquor store on the way home.

I quit drinking two weeks before my 38th birthday and even now I'm sometimes surprised I managed. But I acknowledged the problem and that only I had the power to change it.

I created space to spend an entire day sober, thinking consciously about my drinking and nothing else.

For the first three months I was tired and dehydrated, so I listened to my body, slept more, and drank lots of water. But within two weeks the puffiness in my face reduced. I focused my attention on things I cared about more than drinking. Feeling good became motivating. At three months, I was volunteering at the 2012 Olympics and I felt like an athlete. I wouldn't have missed it for the world. Or a hangover.

Changing my relationship with alcohol was the priority, more important than exercising or eating healthily. I've recently become the fittest I've ever been, but that's a by-product of the work I've done on my emotional development. I've reconnected with my core values and I have the energy to live them.

People used to reinforce my drinking, so I made sure I surrounded myself with people who supported my not-drinking. I had to find my tribe. Most importantly, I told myself that it was possible, that I could do it. And that I already had everything that I needed inside of me— honestly, that's part of why Club Soda exists, because it helps me, too.

MY STORY:
MY DRINKING

THIS SPACE IS FOR YOUR NOTES. THIS SECTION FOCUSES ON PAYING ATTENTION TO YOUR DRINKING AND WHY YOU WANT IT TO CHANGE. JOT DOWN THINGS THAT YOU NOTICE AND ANYTHING ELSE THAT IS HELPFUL TO YOU.

BECOMING MINDFUL—QUESTIONS TO ASK

These notes pages work alongside the prompts across pages 24–27. Complete in the spaces below or copy into your journal or notebook.

WHERE?

Where did I drink alcohol?

Where did I not drink alcohol (if I had the opportunity)?

Where was I when I had more to drink than I wanted to?

WHEN?
When did I drink alcohol?

When did I not drink alcohol (if I had the opportunity)?

When did I drink more than I wanted to?

WHO?
Who did I drink with?

Who did I not drink with (if I had the opportunity)?

Who was I with when I drank more than I wanted to?

WHAT?

What did I drink?

What did I not drink (if I had the opportunity)?

What did I drink when I drank more than I wanted to?

HOW MUCH?

PUTTING IT ALL TOGETHER

What surprises me?

What did I already know that I was failing to admit to myself?

How do I feel about what I have noticed?

What clues does this information give me about how I might change my drinking?

MY DRINKING STORIES

Explore the stories you tell yourself about drinking (see also pages 28–31). Complete below or copy into your journal or notebook.

My caption for this moment
would be ....

My future ....

WEIGHING MY DECISIONS ABOUT DRINKING

Explore the reasons to change your drinking using the decision balance sheet opposite (see also pages 34–35). Complete or copy into your journal or notebook, then tally your scores to see what it reveals.

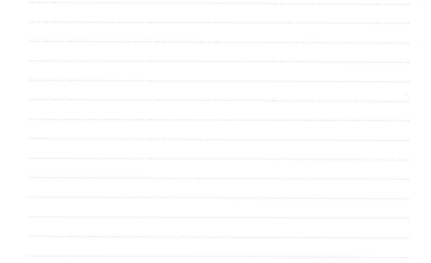

Reasons why	Reasons why not
B + C =	A + D =

ANY OTHER NOTES

MY DECISION BALANCE SHEET	UPSIDES (what will be good, benefits, gains)	DOWNSIDES (what will be difficult, risks, losses)
Staying the same (not changing drinking)	A =	B =
Changing drinking	C =	D =

GETTING STARTED

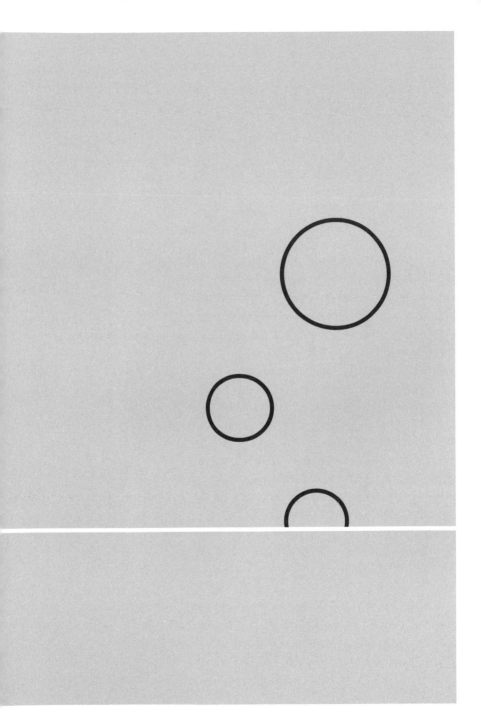

LIVING WITH INTENTION

For too many of us, life simply happens. But we can live differently. We can choose to become active participants instead. As we decide for ourselves, we begin to flourish. We begin to become who we are, to live the life we imagine.

As we first discovered on page 8, **an intention is about committing mindfully to what we want and plan to do**. Such intentions are powerful.

Let's not call these intentions goals, though; goals sound too much like being at work. If you've asked yourself why you want to change your drinking (see page 34), it's likely your answers focused more on how you want to live day by day, how you want to feel about yourself, and who you want to become.

What intentions and goals share in common, however, is that they allow us to articulate clearly what it is that we want. But where goals focus on achieving and getting things, intentions allow us to describe the way in which we want to live, and the type of person that we want to become.

Many of us dream of living differently, but we don't ever say these things out loud. So the dreams remain vague and unfulfilled. Having clear intentions is about being honest with yourself about the need for change, and owning up to your aspirations for your own life.

When we want to live with intention, the key is acting with intention.

Living with intention is about making conscious and deliberate efforts, day by day, to make those dreams a reality. Living with intention means you stop being a spectator and start taking control of your life, changing it for the better.

WHO AM I BECOMING?

Intentions ground you in the here and now.
Intentions help you respond to what you notice.
Intentions support you to become who you are.

Imagine your life in concentric circles. You are at the center, with your thoughts, your feelings, and your body. As you move toward the outer circles, you begin to encounter other people: lovers, partners, children, family, friends. And beyond those closest to you, you find your social life, your working life, and the wider world.

Work

Friends

Family

If you have plenty of space, you could lay circles out on the ground and physically step between them. Or you could just do this in your imagination. As you physically or imaginatively step into each circle, become fully present to who you are in that part of your life, then ask yourself the following:

ME

• Who do I want to become?
• What does it mean for me to live my life well?
• How do I want to feel, to think, and to act?

Take your time over this; be methodical and write everything down—in the notes pages of this chapter (see page 66) or in your journal. If you notice something that intrigues you, stay with it. You are discovering the life you want and starting to put that into words, maybe for the first time.

Begin to focus on your intentions. Then complete this sentence: **I want to be someone who ...**

CHOOSING HOW TO CHANGE

Despite all the social pressures around us and all the urges in us, it's important to remember that drinking isn't compulsory. You can choose whether alcohol has a role to play in the life you imagine.

Consider this: if you knew you didn't have to drink again, are there parts of your life into which you would introduce alcohol? There's no right or wrong answer. It's completely OK if you answer "yes" or "no." It's also OK to want to put certain conditions on that answer: yes, and only in these circumstances; no, but with this exception. Once you have an ideal arrangement in mind, you can test it against reality.

WHAT WILL WORK FOR YOU?

Some Club Soda members talk about not having an off-switch when it comes to drinking. Others have one, but find it doesn't always work.

The off-switch is, of course, a story we tell ourselves about our drinking. We don't have a literal switch inside us that stops us drinking. Scientists of all kinds occasionally go looking for such a device and they get excited to discover a collection of genes, a particular protein, or a behavioral characteristic. But deep down inside we know there's no one single thing.

Our innate sense of how much is too much, and our ability to stop before we reach that point, can change in different circumstances. Our bodies take time to process the alcohol we consume and its effects aren't instant. So, we can drink faster than we get drunk, only realizing we're in trouble when we've already had too much. And some of us appear unable to stop at that point, seemingly determined to drink the house dry or pass out trying.

Noticing your drinking (see pages 24–27) will help you understand what might work for you in reality. Pay attention to the situations in which you drank more than you wanted to, but also those times when you were able to say "no."

So, how will you change? Considering the ideal role you'd like alcohol to play in your life, balanced against the reality of what you know about yourself at this stage, what conclusions will you come to? It's OK to be unsure. You can try something and change your mind. Some people quit drinking, having tried moderation first; others move in the opposite direction, carefully reintroducing alcohol into their lives after a period of abstinence.

You will settle into what works for you. And you can revisit your chosen approach whenever you want.

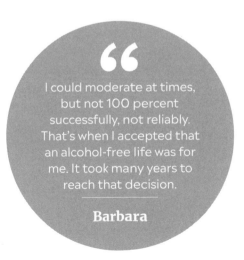

> I could moderate at times, but not 100 percent successfully, not reliably. That's when I accepted that an alcohol-free life was for me. It took many years to reach that decision.
>
> **Barbara**

MAKING PLANS

The act of planning helps us live with intention. In the beginning, daily planning helps. Find time each morning to think through the day. Everything you noticed before about where, when, who with, what, and how much you drink (see pages 24–27) becomes an opportunity to make practical changes. It's a good idea to get down on paper all your thoughts and ideas on this, either in the notes pages (see page 66) or in your notebook or journal.

WHERE?

If you live alone, you can choose whether or not to bring alcohol home with you. If you share your home with someone who drinks, talk to them about your plans—but bear in mind that this change is about you, not them (see page 124).

If you noticed that you mostly drink with others, don't shut yourself away like a hermit. You'll need to navigate social situations and being with people is still good for you. Suggest meeting friends in places where alcohol isn't available or go to the bar but choose a no- or low-alcohol drink instead.

> "
>
> At first, I removed myself from people and places that I found triggering, especially pubs and clubs. Supportive friends met me in restaurants or museums instead.
>
> **Jimmy**

WHEN?

Knowing when you are likely to want to drink means you can plan to control those situations or avoid them altogether. You can switch a Sunday afternoon drinking session into an opportunity for a leisurely walk instead, or steer clear of Thursday night after-work drinks altogether, if that's easier. You don't have to stay anywhere for a moment longer than you want to. There's no shame in escaping to spend time with a good box set.

WHO?

When sharing your plans about changing your drinking with others, not everyone will react well. Defensive people might take your decision as a criticism of them and try to push drinks on you to make themselves feel better. Practice ways to say "no." Good friends will want to support you to live your life well. Be honest and brave in your conversations. You might even inspire them to think about their drinking, too.

WHAT?

You're going to want something else to drink instead and the good news is that we've already made a start on this for you (see pages 138–159). Search local supermarkets and discover what you can buy online. Plan ahead by looking up drinks menus online or make the most of what the bar has to offer by ordering off-menu (see page 144).

HOW MUCH?

If you are alcohol-free, it's easy enough to know you are not drinking alcohol. But how much you drink of other things can matter, too. Dehydration is tiring and makes it harder to make good decisions, so you might want to keep an eye on your fluid intake more generally. And if you replace alcohol in the evening with caffeinated drinks, your sleep could be disrupted.

If you're moderating, for example by choosing to have a specific number of drinks, make a solid plan that you know you can stick to. Start the evening with two nonalcoholic drinks to pace yourself. And drink slowly so you can notice how each drink makes you feel. You might have planned to have two glasses of wine, but you can decide to stop whenever you want.

MEASURING PROGRESS

We forget so much, even when we are paying attention. On our journeys of changing our drinking, we need ways to remind ourselves about what works and what doesn't, so tracking how we're doing is vital. As we enact our plans day by day, and as we grow into the lives we imagine, it's good to be able to look back and see how far we've come. Recording what we notice gives us a way of measuring progress.

Noticing positive progress gives you a reason to celebrate. Take a look at the three things below. Knowing what to notice can help frame how you're measuring your progress. Paying attention to things going in the wrong direction allows you to see that and take action. Either way, continuing to pay attention and measuring your progress will help keep you on track.

WHAT YOU MIGHT NOTICE

There are three kinds of things that you might want to pay attention to.

How your drinking is changing

How you feel

How changing your drinking is changing you

HOW TO TRACK YOUR PROGRESS

To help guide your journey to mindful drinking, each chapter has a notes section at its end. With key questions and prompts, this may be the place for you to jot down your feelings, thoughts, and ideas as you go. Or if you enjoy writing, keep a journal. Tech lovers may prefer the digital approach and there are various apps available that can track many things—from mood and sleep to heart rate and fluid intake. Use whatever helps you notice what matters to you.

If you are using trackers and apps, be sure to download them and start using them now, so you have a baseline before you change your drinking. As you pay attention to what's going on in your world, you'll also be able to see how changing your drinking is creating space for you to flourish.

And check in online, too (joinclubsoda.com). Club Soda members often just share what's happening in their lives and encourage each other to keep going.

How are your plans working out? Are you keeping track of what you're drinking, when, where, and how much (see pages 24–27)?

Because alcohol affects mood, keeping track of how you feel every day is important. Noticing patterns in your emotions can help you avoid drinking when you don't want to, especially if you've been prone to drinking to cope with difficulty.

Sleep, energy, confidence, relationships—all these things can begin to shift over the coming weeks and months; Part 2 reveals how.

OVERCOMING OBSTACLES

It's the little things that trip us up. We can see when the path ahead is blocked by big obstacles. We slow down, assess the options, adjust our plans, and find another way. But it's the tree root, the loose stone, or the uneven path that surprises us and leaves us face down in the dirt. If that happens, then what?

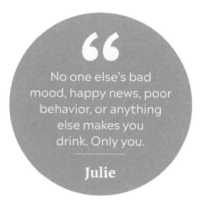

> **❝**
>
> No one else's bad mood, happy news, poor behavior, or anything else makes you drink. Only you.
>
> **Julie**

DREAMS AREN'T ENOUGH

For decades, self-help gurus have said that if you want something enough, it will appear in your life. They've encouraged everyone to visualize their best selves and imagine the happiest possible outcome.

It's true that positive thinking can motivate us to change, but it seems dreams alone aren't enough.

• Because positive thinking stimulates the pleasure centers in our brains, we feel as if we've already achieved something, even though we haven't yet.

• Positive thinking also fails to account for inevitable obstacles, big and small. One way you can make your intentions more effective is by mentally contrasting them with what might go wrong. By actively expecting the obstacles to appear, you can better prepare strategies for them in advance.

That doesn't mean giving up on your intentions; they motivate you to keep going. And just focusing on the obstacles might make you want to give up. So, you need both.

Remember, climbing the mountain requires two things: the mountain and the climb. If you never learn to climb, the mountain remains something you simply admire from afar.

IF-THEN PLANNING

A simple approach that can help you prepare for the little obstacles that you will encounter is "if–then planning." It focuses you on what is most likely to go wrong and helps you figure out how you are going to tackle the problem practically. If–then planning is as simple as saying to yourself: if this happens, then I will do that. It's like a deal you make with your future self.

How if-then planning works best

Here are a few examples that show that making your plans specific is the best way to go.

IF ...	THEN ...
... my friend offers me a drink	... I will politely say "no."
... there's nothing I want to drink at the bar	... I will go home.
... I'm feeling stressed at the end of the day	... I will close my eyes for five minutes and focus on my breathing.
... the kids are annoying me	... I will call a friend.

BELIEVING IN YOURSELF

A healthy measure of self-confidence can supercharge your ability to change your drinking. But for too long too many of us have believed that we are powerless to change. It's time to start believing in yourself.

Fortunately, self-confidence is an attitude that you can develop and strengthen. The more you practice it, the easier it becomes.

Below we share some self-confidence boosters. Consider this a pep talk.

CHANGE ONE THING

One way of building confidence in your ability to change is to look for an easy win. It doesn't have to be related to changing your drinking. Any little niggle that's been bothering you for a while: act on it now. Change the things you can, not the things you can't. Celebrate your small victories extravagantly.

BEWARE OF COMPARISONS

When you compare your insides to other people's outsides, you will always come up short. Your experience of your own inner world, in which you are acutely aware of your worries, faults, and failings, is always going to compare badly to the outward appearance of another person's life. But remember that you can't ever know what life is really like for them. If you could experience another person's life for even a moment, you would realize that they, too, are making it up as they go along. What you see is just a projection of their confidence.

 3

FAKE IT TILL YOU MAKE IT

For once, this is something that the self-help industry gets absolutely right. Building self-confidence can work from the outside in: when you act as if you know what you are doing, you begin to feel more confident. Standing straighter, speaking up, and connecting with others are simple ways of showing others that you are not afraid to take up space in the world.

 4

BEFRIEND YOUR INNER CRITIC

There is a part of you that has a forensic gaze, that fearlessly tells the truth, and that easily distinguishes between good and bad: say "hello" to your inner critic. For too long, your inner critic's energy has been turned against you. They have tried so hard to make sure you are safe by keeping you in your place. But you don't need this kind of "protection" any more. You're ready to face the world as the person you are becoming.

You can thank your inner critic for trying to look after you. And then you can make them your ally, drawing on all that fearsome independence as your own.

AVOIDING PERFECTIONISM

Things will and do go wrong. That's life. But for perfectionists that is a hard fact to accept. Perfectionism makes us prone to setting unrealistically high standards. We tend to see the world in black and white. So, when faced with challenges, we can lose all sense of proportion and experience any minor setbacks as major catastrophes.

The pain of the imperfection we feel in ourselves may be a reason that some of us drink more than we want to. When we're changing our drinking, perfectionism can hold us back.

FORGET STANDARDS

Remember, changing your drinking isn't about achieving goals. If you live your intentions day by day, you'll begin to become aware of the unrealistic standards you've been imposing on yourself. Pay attention especially to anything you feel you should do.

Stop striving to be who you think you should be. Give yourself space to become who you are.

BEYOND BLACK AND WHITE

Black-and-white thinking is a particular issue if you choose an alcohol-free life. Many people who stop drinking begin counting days of sobriety on day one. As the number of days goes up, so does your self-confidence. But this approach might store up an ever-growing risk.

Because ... what happens when you slip up? If your view is a black-and-white one, you'll focus on the moment of failure and reset your counter all the way back to day one. But do you really need to do that?

NOT A CATASTROPHE

The night when it all goes wrong is only a catastrophe if you let it be one. As you nurse a hangover the next day, try to keep things in perspective (once your brain is able to function). Notice what happened. Revisit your intentions. Adjust your plans for the next time, if you need to.

Nobody is perfect. Even with the clearest intentions and the strongest plans, things will still go wrong sometimes. Slip-ups will happen. Every mistake is a chance to learn. No mistake is a catastrophe. Perfectionism can paralyze you. But don't let your desire to fix everything stop you changing something. Start where you stand, then keep going, step by step.

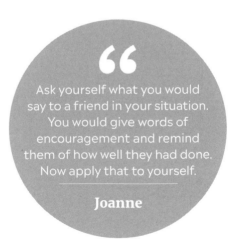

Ask yourself what you would say to a friend in your situation. You would give words of encouragement and remind them of how well they had done. Now apply that to yourself.

Joanne

YOU ARE READY

The first two chapters are all about getting ready. Getting you to this moment.

Are you ready to change your drinking? Then it's time to choose when to begin. It doesn't have to be a significant date, such as New Year's Day. In fact, you might want to choose an ordinary day on which not much happens.

Now, it's just the final preparations for the big day, a bit like packing before a vacation or the last run through of a checklist—you need to plan ahead and assemble your survival kit.

REVIEW AND PLANNING

First, take time to remind yourself of your intentions. Why do you want to change your drinking? Who do you want to become? And what role does alcohol play in the life you imagine?

Find the intentions you wrote down before and display them somewhere you'll see them often—as a continual nudge in the right direction. Remind yourself how you want this sentence to finish:

> **I want to be someone who ...**

Make a rock-solid plan for the first few days, particularly considering where and when you normally drink, and who you drink with. Again, keep notes. Create some if–then plans to get you through the tricky moments that may come up. Remember, it's OK to avoid things rather than trying to control them. Escape is always an option.

You'll have probably already decided how you'll measure progress (see page 54) so make sure whatever kinds you're using are ready to go. Now might be a good time to reflect on how you are feeling, before you begin.

It's a good idea to go out of your way to make these early days as easy as possible. And remind yourself that it's OK if you don't get it right first time.

YOUR SURVIVAL KIT

The second type of preparation is entirely practical and helps you to practice being kind to yourself. As well as your recently started journal (or apps) to track your progress, gather some things that will nurture you through the first few days; we'd suggest:

- something to drink instead of alcohol (see page 144–159)
- healthy and nutritious foods that are easy to prepare
- some sweet treats to deal with sugar cravings
- something to pamper yourself with
- a reward to celebrate the progress you make.

Do resist the urge to drink the house dry the night before. You really don't want to begin this phase by nursing the hangover from hell.

YOU'VE GOT THIS

We won't wish you good luck. Becoming a mindful drinker isn't a matter of luck. It's about:

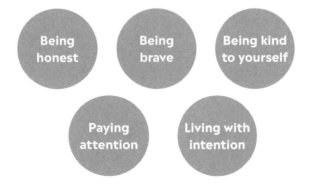

Being honest

Being brave

Being kind to yourself

Paying attention

Living with intention

ANJA HAS BEEN CHANGING HER
DRINKING OVER THE LAST TWO YEARS

HOW I CHANGED MY DRINKING: **ANJA'S STORY**

I've worked in hospitality—behind bars and in breweries—for years; it's a dangerous industry. You're surrounded by booze and nobody warns you: "Careful how you use that stuff." When life gets tough, drink is there—usually cheap or free. It's easy to hide a complicated relationship with alcohol behind being a connoisseur. We drink for the taste, so it can't be problematic, right?

Except I was so unhappy that I was barely functioning. I couldn't make decisions, I barely ate, and I didn't nourish relationships because I was working constantly. Work was breaking me and I wanted to disappear. It was a toxic environment.

I was facing redundancy and I didn't have it in me to fight it. I drank because it was there. It was almost daily, to congratulate myself on surviving and to numb the thought of doing it again tomorrow. Not spectacular amounts, but I didn't like the habit I was forming.

An impossible challenge seemed the only thing to facilitate the transformation I wanted in myself. I signed up for Marathon des Sables, a 156-mile race in the Sahara. I told everyone. I knew they'd think I couldn't and I knew that meant I would! I trained hard and cutting down came naturally and fairly easily. This was also when I started working with Club Soda, thinking and talking about alcohol a lot and discovering a world of alcohol-free drinks.

But before the race, I felt ill. On returning home, I was diagnosed with tuberculosis. It had begun eating holes in my lungs. Treatment sent my liver function into decline and I was placed in isolation for 11 days. I spent a year on brutal medication. I was very unwell and I barely drank, probably more due to circumstances than mindfulness.

My illness might have been a setback but it also allowed me to slow down. I'm cultivating a better life now. I still work in the beer industry but feel I'm edging my way out. That's scary. I've dedicated 11 years of my career to it. But the brave choice is seeking things that bring joy, and I've always wanted to be brave.

I'd been a talented pianist. Creative things were once part of my identity, but I'd let them become things I used to do. I'm about to take an extended break from drinking, for the pure indulgence of time to reflect and reconnect with those creative things as acts of self-care. I don't know if I'll ever quit completely; I'm a mindful drinker in progress.

MY STORY:
MY BEGINNINGS

THIS SPACE IS FOR YOUR NOTES ON YOUR INTENTIONS, PLANS, AND PROGRESS. JOT DOWN THINGS THAT YOU NOTICE AND ANYTHING ELSE THAT IS HELPFUL TO YOU AS YOU START YOUR MINDFUL DRINKING JOURNEY

DISCOVERING MY INTENTIONS – WHO AM I BECOMING?

These notes pages work alongside the prompts across pages 48–57. Complete in the spaces below or copy into your journal or notebook.

Who do I want to become?

What does it mean for me to live my life well?

How do I want to feel, to think, and to act?

I want to be someone who...

MY PLAN TO CHANGE MY DRINKING

What practical changes will I make to my drinking?

Where?

When?

Who with?

What?

How much?

MY IF–THEN PLANS

As I change my drinking, there will be obstacles to overcome. This is how I'll tackle them:

IF...	THEN...

ANY OTHER NOTES

Being a mindful drinker changes more than how you feel about alcohol. Over time, other parts of your life will begin to change, too—your physical health, your mood, and your relationships with other people.

Many of these changes will feel positive. Some good things may take a while to emerge; other changes will be immediate. But there might be challenges as well.

We've packed this part of the book with our collective wisdom so you know what to expect and what to do.

If things get tough, don't give up. It'll all be OK in the end. If it's not OK, it's not the end.

And if you need help, reach out. You're sure to find another Club Soda member who has been where you are.

PART 2
CHANGING

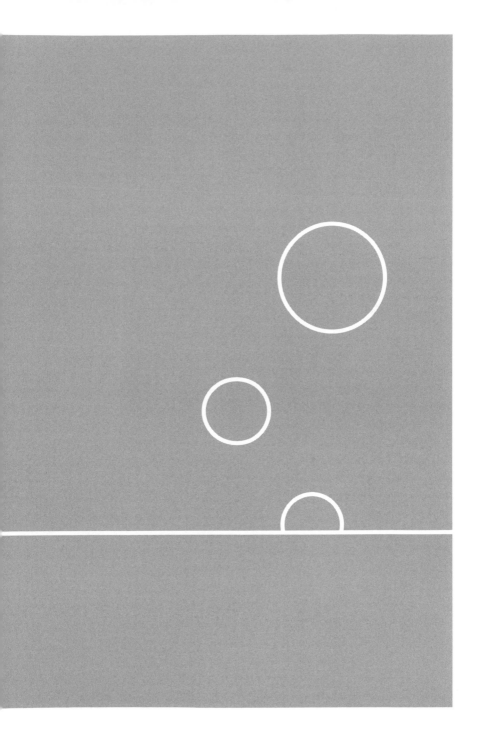

DRINKING AND YOUR HEALTH

YOUR BODY // NUTRITION // ENERGY //
SLEEP // BUTCH'S STORY // MY STORY: MY BODY

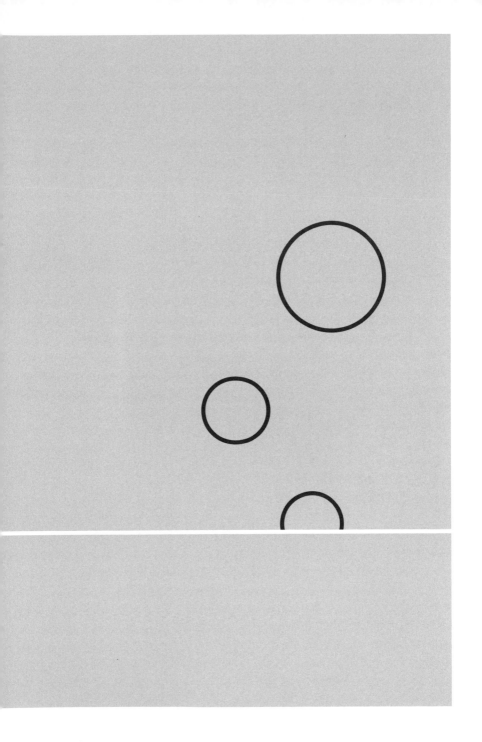

YOUR BODY

When we become mindful drinkers, our bodies benefit immediately. One of the obvious and immediate upsides of changing our drinking is that we eliminate hangovers. Drinking-related headaches, dehydration, nausea, and diarrhea will become distant memories.

As mindful drinkers, many of us will experience changes in how we eat (see page 78), in how energetic we feel (see page 80), and in how well we sleep (see page 82). These are big issues for lots of us, so we've dedicated whole sections on what to expect and what to do.

Other changes are as individual as we are: our skin may become less puffy; period pain might lessen; hot flashes may be easier to deal with. Over the coming weeks and months, keep track of what's happening physically, so you can see how your body is responding to this change.

There's also a lot going on beneath the surface of our skin that we can't directly feel or see. Our bodies feel the benefits of reducing the amount we drink, especially if we have regular days that are alcohol-free and avoid heavy drinking sessions. Spending longer periods without alcohol frees our livers to start shedding the extra fat cells they have accumulated. Our blood pressure can start to reduce. Our cholesterol levels can begin to normalize. Our risk of cancer and heart disease can diminish.

So, with so many obvious benefits of mindful drinking, why on earth do we ever believe that drinking alcohol is good for us?

QUESTION EVERYTHING YOU READ (EVEN THIS!)

One of the stories you might have told yourself about drinking (see pages 28 and 42) is that alcohol is "good for you." There are endless headlines about the upsides of alcohol that support this belief: whether it's scientists discovering that champagne "prevents dementia," a new study claiming that red wine "protects against heart disease," or researchers saying that beer is "packed with vital vitamins." You might have taken them at face value before, but approach such news stories with a healthy skepticism. Many scientists diligently report their studies only to find details exaggerated or even wilfully misinterpreted. We all tend to look for evidence to back up what we want to believe, and that's as true for health journalists as it is for us.

All the apparent benefits of alcohol can be gained in other ways. Other people might cling to any reason, however unlikely, to keep drinking. But you're not "other people" any more, and you know better than to blindly trust everything you read in the papers or online.

PAY ATTENTION TO YOUR BODY

Take time to regularly check in with how your body feels. Sit quietly where you won't be disturbed and scan your body—by this we mean, bring your attention to each part of your body in turn. Some people like to start at the toes and work up the body, bit by bit; others like to do the reverse, starting off at the head. Whichever direction, notice what's going on. Then ask yourself:

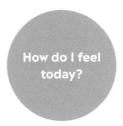

How do I feel today?

You will know better than anyone how you normally feel, and you will be able to sense changes if you pay regular attention. Whether it's aches and pains, physical discomfort, or other symptoms that emerge, if something is bothering you, don't ignore it. Take an interest in your well-being and look after yourself. And if you need extra support from a health care professional, seek out help.

NUTRITION

We do not eat well when we are drunk. Alcohol simultaneously increases our appetite and decreases our ability to make good food choices. Some of us, in fact, actively avoid food so we can drink more without gaining weight or drink so much that we forget to eat at all, while others drink through huge boozy lunches or alone with chips on the sofa. Drinking more than we want to might cover up the troubled nature of our relationship with food.

As you change what you drink, you can begin to adjust how you eat as well. All your mindful drinking skills—particularly paying attention and acting with intention—will help you if you want to change your eating habits, too.

LOSING WEIGHT

Ounce for ounce, alcohol is one of the most energy-dense substances you can consume. As a mindful drinker, you might expect to lose weight; it might have been a reason to change your drinking. Sadly, it's not that straightforward. Your beer belly grew slowly, so you shouldn't expect it to disappear overnight.

As you change your drinking, you may find your appetite fluctuates. Sugar cravings are common, but this is nothing to worry about in the short term. You don't have to change everything at once, and reducing your sugar consumption is something you can tackle when you're ready.

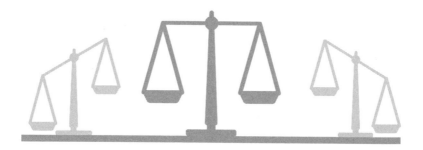

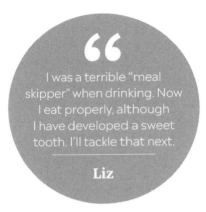

> "
> I was a terrible "meal skipper" when drinking. Now I eat properly, although I have developed a sweet tooth. I'll tackle that next.
>
> **Liz**

Rather than depriving yourself through dieting, focus on foods that nourish you and support your well-being. As you change your drinking, your taste buds will reawaken. Now's a great opportunity to start experimenting, trying new recipes, and noticing new and old flavors.

And bear in mind that numbers on the bathroom scale aren't as important as how you feel in your own skin. In an image-obsessed society, it's a radical act to love yourself just as you are.

RESTORING YOUR BODY

Drinking can leave you deficient in many vitamins and minerals. That's not just because you might make poor food choices, but because alcohol can prevent and inhibit your body's absorption and use of nutrients. B vitamins, for example, are vital to keep nerve cells healthy, but they are the first to be washed out of your body when it is flooded with booze. Everything from vitamin A to zinc can take a hit from drinking.

As you change your drinking, you'll improve your gut's ability to absorb nutrients from the food you eat. So help your gut out by eating nutritious meals. In the short term, vitamin and mineral supplements can help, but for your longer-term health shift to eating a varied and nourishing diet.

ENERGY

Many of us who have been drinking mindfully for a while find ourselves with fresh stores of energy and renewed enthusiasm for life. But it doesn't happen overnight. In the early days it's common to feel wiped out, particularly if you go completely alcohol-free.

As you begin to experience the benefits of mindful drinking, you may also start to realize how much your body has been through. In terms of metabolism, alcohol consistently goes to the front of the line; your body is used to prioritizing alcohol over other functions, so it takes time to adjust to its absence. Drinking might have left you sleep-deprived, since alcohol affects critical parts of the sleep cycle (see page 82). And a whole bunch of avoided emotional issues might be starting to catch up with you, too.

Energy will come, but for now, prioritize self-care. Remember the survival kit you put together when you were getting ready (see page 63)? Now's the time to use it. And, remember, sleep is your friend—your body is hard at work healing itself while you're snoozing.

As your energy returns, you'll suddenly notice that you have time on your hands. Without hangovers, weekends are yours and even week days seem longer. How best to use this renewed energy? See opposite for a couple of ideas.

QUIT SMOKING

If you don't smoke tobacco, or you quietly quit alongside changing your drinking, you can skip ahead to "Move your body," opposite. But if you are still smoking, this next section is especially for you.

As with drinking, we're not going to lecture you. We know that quitting smoking is hard. But smoking increases cravings for alcohol (see page 188), so if you find yourself struggling often with the urge to drink, you would do yourself a favor by getting the help you need to tackle your tobacco habit.

Many of us who successfully change our drinking find smoking much harder to deal with, so you're not alone. The health benefits associated with quitting smoking are too numerous to detail here, but it will also give your energy levels a significant boost. That's why we mention it.

Lots of the techniques in this book can be applied to smoking, but we're not experts in this area. Seek specialist advice and the support you need.

MOVE YOUR BODY

A drinking life is a sedentary life. As your energy levels begin to recover, you can give yourself an extra boost by getting moving. It may seem counterintuitive, but expending energy on exercise does improve energy levels. Physical activity could also help you feel better about yourself, improving your self-esteem and your mood, and—if you exercise with other people—it could give you a welcome new social focus, too.

If you've been inactive for a while, the idea of exercise can be intimidating. So start small. You don't need to begin training for a marathon (though some Club Soda members do). Find ways of moving your body that you enjoy: walking, dancing, swimming, lifting weights, yoga, running. And don't forget—sex counts as exercise, too (see page 122).

SPEND TIME IN NATURE

A drinking life is often an indoor life. Yet, a world awaits outside your windows. Spending just a few hours each week in nature is good for your physical health and is scientifically proven to support your emotional well-being, too. Many people report the restorative and energy-giving benefits of being in places where nature reigns and the human world recedes. Time outdoors doesn't need to involve camping off-grid or weeks of hiking. Your local park is just as good.

Immersing yourself in nature can be a great way to practice paying attention, too. Notice what's happening around you, breathe deeply, and relax.

SLEEP

Drinking alcohol keeps us from sleeping well. Unfortunately, in the short-term, changing our drinking can do exactly the same thing. Sleep disturbance is such a common side-effect when we change our drinking, it's one of the reasons people most often cite if they start drinking again. But there are good ways to deal with sleepless nights, and any such issues soon improve.

ALCOHOL AND SLEEP

If you rely on alcohol's sedative qualities to get you to sleep, you will also know the downsides: waking up but not feeling refreshed, needing to pee frequently, feeling dehydrated, your heart pounding. Drinking makes you dream less and snore more. You don't so much sleep as pass out.

Things will change, but there's no need to fret about sleeping while alcohol-free. Before long, your body will adjust to alcohol-free bedtimes.

LETTING SLEEP HAPPEN

Worrying about sleep can keep you awake. Remember, sleep doesn't require effort. It will arrive when you stop trying to make it happen. That said, there are some practical things you can do to encourage sleep to happen.

- Set regular times for going to bed and for getting up—good sleep hygiene, as it's known, is one of the keys to great sleep.
- Watch your caffeine intake and choose soothing bedtime drinks, such as herbal teas or hot milk.
- Avoid screens before bedtime. Bright lights, particularly blue wavelengths, can suppress the production of melatonin, an essential sleep hormone.
- Take a warm bath.
- Write a to-do list for the next day before bed if you are prone to worrying.
- Keep your bedroom dark, tidy, quiet, and cool.

And if you still don't fall asleep, don't lie there worrying and checking the clock. Get up and find a quiet corner to sit. Read a book or listen to relaxing music until you feel tired enough to doze off.

It's worth keeping in mind that eight hours of sleep is just a rule of thumb. If you wake up feeling refreshed, you've had enough sleep.

DRINKING DREAMS

Dreams in which you're drinking happen, and they are normal, even years after you've changed! Whatever occurs in your dream, be reassured that it isn't an omen that you're about to fall off the wagon. That said, it might be a nudge to pay attention to what's going on in your inner world, particularly if it makes you aware of cravings (see page 188) or ambivalence (see page 190).

Write about your dream in your journal (or note it in your app or tracker). Write in the present tense and focus on your emotions: "In my dream, I am … In my dream, I feel …." Your dream might tempt you to romanticize the past, so use the opportunity to remind yourself of your intentions (see pages 48 and 66).

> **"**
> I stopped ignoring all the sensible advice people gave me—reduced screen time; regular bedtime; hot baths; a cool, dark room. It has been transformative.
>
> **Anja**

BUTCH IS A TRUCK DRIVER WHOSE
HEALTH HAS IMPROVED SINCE QUITTING

HOW I CHANGED MY DRINKING: **BUTCH'S STORY**

When people ask: "What is the one thing that stopping drinking has given you?" I always say "inner peace." True joy comes from within.

At my worst, I drank an awful lot. I was drinking almost a bottle of vodka a day. I'd wake up hungover, then make a drink to relieve it. I'd get the shakes, I couldn't sign my name sometimes. It was horrible.

It's so easy to get pulled in because when you think about it we drink for everything. We drink to celebrate, to commiserate, at sporting events, at weddings. It's never-ending.

I've been seeing my doctor every year for 27 years. I'd have my blood work done and my liver enzymes would be elevated. He would ask, and of course, I would lie. Every year it got worse. I was worried about my health and I always felt lousy. My stomach caused the most trouble. It was upset a lot.

I'd tried to stop several times and always fallen flat on my face. I remember telling my wife, "I joined Club Soda, I think it's going to help me at least moderate my drinking if I don't quit completely." I saw the skepticism on her face. She'd heard it all before. But I haven't had a drink since. The support group is what I lacked before.

Eventually, I told my doctor: "I was drinking more than I told you." He said: "I know that! You think you can fool your doctor, but we see it all. Your physical appearance even shows it."

My emotions now are true emotions. When I'm happy or sad or grieving, it's not alcohol-fueled. Even when I cry it feels good because it's not caused by substances.

I do more than I used to. My wife and I have been taking short trips. We see magnificent places that we never would have visited during my drinking career. Last weekend we drove up to a beautiful spot in the mountains with a waterfall. We hiked to the base of the falls just to stand and feel the mist blow against our faces. I never would have done that before.

My old drinking buddies had a bet as to how long I would last. The longest that someone suggested was six weeks. Nobody has collected yet. Nobody will collect. I use that to motivate me.

I look back at all the years I've wasted because I was drunk, and the time I could've spent with my family. Everyone makes mistakes and I feel as though I've been forgiven for mine.

MY STORY:

MY BODY

THIS SPACE IS FOR YOUR NOTES ON YOUR PHYSICAL HEALTH, ENERGY LEVELS, EATING HABITS, AND SLEEP. ALSO KEEP A NOTE OF THINGS THAT YOU NOTICE AND ANYTHING ELSE THAT IS HELPFUL TO YOU.

These notes pages work alongside pages 76–83. Complete in the spaces below or copy into your journal or notebook.

CHECKING IN WITH MY BODY

Use the charts opposite and on the next page to record how your physical health changes as you move along your mindful drinking journey—both the good and the bad. How often you check in with your body is up to you, but remember that such changes take time so it's better to pace your checks across a few weeks rather than days.

CHECK IN WITH YOUR BODY	Positive changes	Negative changes
Nutrition		
Energy		
Sleep		

CHECK IN WITH YOUR BODY	Positive changes	Negative changes
Nutrition		
Energy		
Sleep		

CHECK IN WITH YOUR BODY	Positive changes	Negative changes
Nutrition		
Energy		
Sleep		

DRINKING AND YOUR MOOD

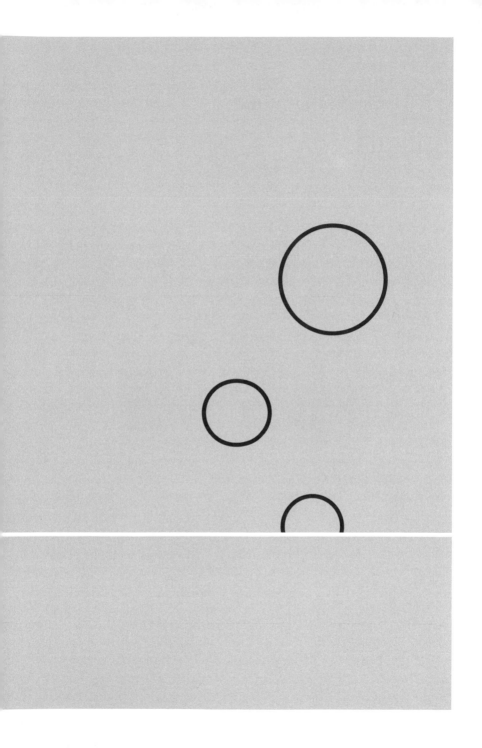

FEELING GOOD

Feeling good feels good. Feelings of calm, contentment, love, and happiness make the world a better place. When we feel good we expand our awareness of the world, we cope better, and we take stressful situations in stride. Feeling good improves our personal and working relationships. And one good feeling so often sparks another.

For some of us, drinking is a shortcut to feeling good. One thing that might hold us back from becoming mindful drinkers is the worry that without alcohol in our lives our happy feelings are going to disappear. Do we even know how to be happy?

TWO TYPES OF HAPPINESS

Positive psychologists identify two types of happiness.

- **Hedonic happiness** This comes when we increase pleasure and reduce pain; it's largely a short-term feeling and happens moment by moment.
- **Eudaemonic happiness** This centers on the kind of positive feelings that come from fulfilment and a sense of purpose in life—a longer-term view.

Drinking can increase hedonic happiness, but it's all too easy to find ourselves drinking ever more to chase the same short-term pleasures, which can seriously compromise our eudaemonic happiness. That's not a good thing.

Let's be clear. Living the life you imagine and putting alcohol in its place is about eudaemonic happiness. But that doesn't mean you have to sacrifice hedonic happiness. You need both types of happiness in your life.

THE PURSUIT OF PLEASURE

Pleasure is the key to hedonic happiness, and seeking it immerses us in the world of our senses. Make an effort daily to notice what brings you pleasure. Keep a list and come back to it over time. Here are some ideas to get you started.

- **Touch** Physical contact with other consenting humans can be intensely pleasurable. Learn to hug, find a dance partner, or enjoy a massage.
- **Taste** Changing your drinking tweaks your taste buds, so savor the flavors. There's pleasure not just in sweetness, but in salt, sour, bitter, and umami as well.
- **Smell** What do freshly cut flowers, cinnamon rolls, or old books bring to mind? Smells are powerful shortcuts to happy memories.
- **Hearing** Music can powerfully shift emotions. Natural soundscapes (away from human-made noise) can reconnect you with the world so you can enjoy its calm pleasures—whether that's listening to birdsong, the rustling of leaves in the wind, or the rain.
- **Sight** All sorts of sights are happy, from faces of loved ones to views of special places. Add happy pictures to your fridge and desk and digital versions to your phone and computer as a screen saver.

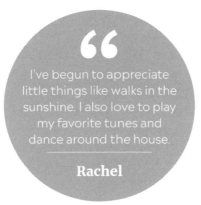

I've begun to appreciate little things like walks in the sunshine. I also love to play my favorite tunes and dance around the house.

Rachel

SADNESS

From childhood, many of us have been taught to "handle" some of our strongest emotions by not dealing with them at all. Nice girls don't get angry. Brave boys don't cry. And nobody is allowed to feel sad for very long. Sound familiar? Instead, we are simply supposed to put all our troublesome feelings away in a box marked "bad."

As we become adults, some of us turn that box into a liquor cabinet. We drink to numb ourselves, pretending the box isn't there as we sit on its lid. Sometimes the box springs open and everything comes rushing out. Regretful hangovers are spent busily stuffing everything back in.

The rich diversity of strong emotions in that box is our birthright as human beings. It's not just drinking that robs us of this incredible gift; it's the culture we live in, too.

OPENING THE BOX

Dealing with our strongest emotions can be hard at first, especially if, like many people, we have been taught that all such feelings should be avoided and if we've been drinking to ignore them.

One of the first emotions we might find when we open the box is sadness. Sadness has many causes:

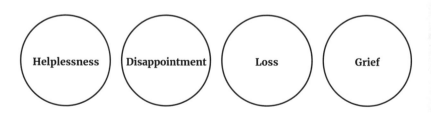

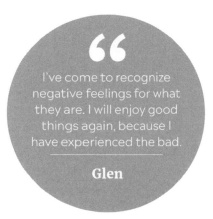

> **"**
> I've come to recognize
> negative feelings for what
> they are. I will enjoy good
> things again, because I
> have experienced the bad.
>
> **Glen**

There's much about the current state of the world that can make us sad. Plus, we might feel sad about our lives. In a society filled with shiny, happy people, sadness can make us feel especially uncomfortable. We put sadness in the box because we don't know quite what to do with it. We are so intent on cheering ourselves up, we forget to ask what sadness might be good for.

EMBRACING SADNESS

Sadness helps show us the parts of our lives that we want to change. It gives us space and time to be kind to ourselves (remember, those three attitudes from page 23—be honest, be brave, and be kind to yourself?). Instead of hurrying to make your sadness go away, how would it be if you embraced it, even welcomed it into your life?

Feeling sad is a normal human experience. So write in your journal, sing sad songs, and have a good cry. Treat yourself kindly and accept your feelings just as they are. If you're keeping track of your moods, you'll notice ups and downs. Find supportive people who will listen without judgment. And if your feelings are beyond your ability to cope with them, seek professional help. There are gifts in the darkness, if you are brave enough to find them.

STRESS

Stress hormones raise our heart rate, increase our breathing, and make us sweat. In response to threats, these hormones get us ready to tackle the threat head-on, run away, or stay as still as possible. We cannot control that physical fight, flight, or freeze response, but we can change how we feel about it.

> **Sources of stress are all around us. Stress affects our moods, but it starts as chemical reactions deep within our bodies.**

Think about roller coasters. If you enjoy them, you'll know the exhilaration as you hurtle upside down around a corner, holding on, and screaming. Your body at that moment is experiencing extreme physical stress. You get off the ride and find yourself shaking (as the hormones flood your body). But instead of causing distress, the feelings in your body are intensely pleasurable.

Once you notice these physical sensations in your body, you can begin to choose how you emotionally respond to them. For instance, is that knot in your stomach really anxiety? Or is it simply a feeling of digestive discomfort that will pass with time? Sweaty palms and a dry mouth don't have to feel like stress. You can just notice what is going on in your body as physical sensations, nothing more.

STRESS RELIEF BEYOND THE BOTTLE

Alcohol does indeed work as a short-term stress-reliever, but there's much more going on when you have a stiff drink to unwind. Team drinks at the end of a stressful workday are also about social connection. The first glass of wine at home is also a moment of calm in a safe environment. But such positive stress-relievers—bonding, refocusing, and self-care—are yours to claim even without a drink in your hand. Breathing techniques, meditation, and walking can also help you relax and ride out the physical sensations of stress. They take practice, but over time they become automatic responses, much like drinking may once have been.

Track your stress levels. Notice certain situations and events that feel particularly difficult. Take notes about how you respond, and pay attention to what works and what doesn't work to help you feel calm.

BUILDING RESILIENCE

You might not be able to change the causes of stress in your life, but you can develop your ability to respond well to stress. Building resilience starts with a commitment to look after yourself. Eating well, getting enough sleep, and moving your body are great stress-busters. As you begin to feel better about yourself, you can begin to tackle the sources of stress in your life. You can't change everything, but you can change how you respond to anything.

REDUCING STRESS

If you are particularly troubled by long-term stress, you might want to explore whether mindfulness-based stress reduction (MBSR) could help you. This structured program incorporates many of the things you've already learned through changing your drinking—such as paying attention, treating yourself kindly, and learning to react less emotionally to your experiences. MBSR has been shown to have positive benefits for people suffering long-term stress, as well as anxiety and depression.

MBSR is often conducted face-to-face over eight weeks in group classes, but you can also find resources and support online.

ANXIETY

From generalized worry to full-blown panic attacks, all of us experience anxiety at some point in our lives. Alcohol is at best a quick and dirty fix for anxiety, but still many of us come to rely on it.

To understand why that doesn't work and why it might actually make things worse, we need to explore how alcohol affects our brains.

ALCOHOL'S UPS AND DOWNS

How is it that some of us tend to fall asleep when we've had too much to drink, while others of us get into aggressive fights?

Although alcohol has been studied extensively, its effects on the brain are incredibly complex and not completely understood. Fortunately, you don't need a degree in neuroscience to understand drinking's ups and downs.

First, the downs: alcohol is a depressant. This doesn't mean that alcohol makes you depressed. Rather, it means that alcohol inhibits some of your brain's functions. It's this sedating effect of alcohol that relaxes you and—depending on how much you drink—makes you sleepy and uncoordinated.

Next, the ups: alcohol is also a stimulant. It creates a pain-killing endorphin high, like opiate drugs do. Drinking increases levels of dopamine, a neurotransmitter linked to reward and pleasure. It also triggers a temporary boost in serotonin, a brain chemical linked with the regulation of mood, appetite, and sleep.

There's another stimulation, too, that's not quite so pleasurable, even in the short-term. Alcohol prompts the release of adrenaline and noradrenaline, which are associated with anxiety and stress.

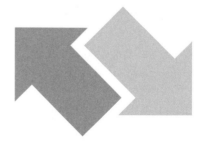

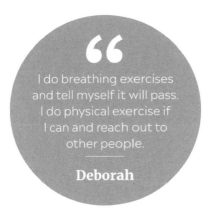

I do breathing exercises and tell myself it will pass. I do physical exercise if I can and reach out to other people.

Deborah

As with other drugs, there's a low that follows alcohol's high, and it's not just because you have a hangover. Your brain chemistry is readjusting, too. This comedown from alcohol can heighten anxiety, and not just due to worries about what might have happened when you were drunk. Alcohol worsens anxiety.

LIVING WITH ANXIETY

So, as you become a mindful drinker, you may find that your anxiety naturally begins to wane. But it's good to begin to learn how to live with anxiety in your day-to-day life. As well as all the usual good things you can do for yourself—eating well and getting enough sleep—here are some specific tips:

- **Talk to others about what's worrying you**. Be specific. Other people can help you put your anxiety into perspective.
- **Get out of your head and into your body**. Consciously moving will help you unfreeze if anxiety is paralyzing. Stand up, stretch, and stamp your feet.
- **Try grounding techniques.** Notice what's around you: five things you can see, four that you can hear, three you can feel (shoes on your feet, not your emotions), two you can smell, and, finally, one thing you can taste.

BOREDOM

Boredom won't kill us, but dealing with it badly really could. Our cultural discomfort with boredom is extreme. Remember the long boring Sunday afternoons you experienced as a child? We've built a hyperstimulated world to try and make boredom impossible. In the face of all the information and entertainment that surrounds us, it can feel as if we have no excuse to be bored.

Boredom does happen, in part, because of what's going on around us. But boredom also happens inside in our brains.

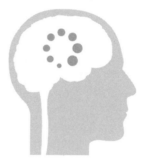

Those of us who are particularly prone to feelings of boredom are more likely to have naturally lower levels of dopamine—the brain's pleasure chemical. We're also more likely to misuse substances. Many of us chase the buzz of alcohol to stave off boredom. We might also use other drugs, take bigger risks, and put ourselves in real danger, all for a dopamine hit to alleviate the boredom.

THE SECRET JOYS OF BOREDOM

When you change your drinking, you might be confronted by boredom. Worse still, unkind people might even tell you that you have become boring. Remind yourself that this says more about them than you. You might even begin to notice how dull and repetitive very drunk people can be.

If you are prone to boredom, that might be a gift. Boredom can push you out of your comfort zone and propel you to explore the world. Some of your boredom may result from how your brain works, but your environment matters, too. A change of scenery really is good for you.

Not drinking means you have more time and money on your hands, as well as increasing amounts of energy (see page 80). So start trying new things. There's so much to discover about yourself and the things you enjoy. And it's OK to be as obsessive about new interests as you were about drinking. Be kind to your novelty- and reward-seeking brain.

As you begin to live the life you imagine and act with intention (see page 48), you will find new ways to pass the time.

And paying attention beats boredom hands down. As you become more mindful, you will find your environment inherently less boring, because you'll notice so much more. And as you feel increasingly comfortable with who you are, you'll also discover that boredom matters less anyway. You will become happier spending time in your own company.

Who knows, you might even discover the secret joys of long, boring Sunday afternoons.

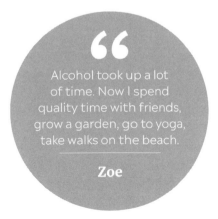

> Alcohol took up a lot of time. Now I spend quality time with friends, grow a garden, go to yoga, take walks on the beach.
>
> **Zoe**

HALT

There are some feelings that are so associated with the urge to drink, they are often turned into an acronym: HALT.

When you are hit out of nowhere by the urge to have a drink, it's useful to ask yourself the following:

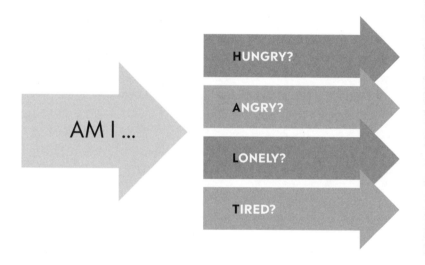

We can answer these questions at a purely practical level.

- **H**unger is a prompt to eat.
- **A**nger is an encouragement to express our feelings.
- **L**oneliness is a cue that we need connection with others.
- **T**iredness is a signal to rest.

Putting these practical needs first will help you avoid the urge to drink.

It's strange, though. None of these states has anything to do with alcohol. So why do we think that drinking will help us solve them?

OUR DEEPEST NEEDS

If we use alcohol to meet any of our emotional needs, we can come to rely on it for all of them. This doesn't happen right away; we learn to depend on drinking over time and with repetition. We don't have our first drink thinking, "this will cure my loneliness." But bit by bit, drinking can fill in the gaps that are left when our feelings are stuck in the box (see page 94).

As you start to explore the emotions you've been hiding away, you might notice that you've been drinking to try to meet some of your deepest needs. Of course, it's never really worked, and now you've changed your drinking, those needs are all still there.

GOING DEEPER WITH HALT

HALT isn't just a summary of reasons for drinking (as opposite); approached differently, you can use this neat acronym to help you acknowledge your deepest needs. Be warned, this is not a day one activity. Do this when you are ready, when you feel emotionally strong, and when you are well-supported.

Then, and only then, ask yourself the following:

- **Hunger** What am I hungry for in life? What do I long for? What needs have I left unmet for too long?
- **Anger** What frustrations are holding me back? What's inside me that wants to be expressed? What pain am I carrying that's weighing me down?
- **Loneliness** What do I need to do to become happy in my own company? How can I meet my desire for connection? What do I want from the relationships in my life?
- **Tiredness** How am I meeting my need for rest and self-care? What am I tired of, that I'm ready to let go of? What do I need to stop, so that I can become who I am?

JACK HAS CHANGED HIS DRINKING
AND IMPROVED HIS MENTAL HEALTH

HOW I CHANGED MY DRINKING: **JACK'S STORY**

When I first started working, I wanted to be the world's best bartender. I set myself a goal to become International Bartender of the Year. I achieved that goal at the age of 23, at a bar I set up with my business partner in New York. Success came quickly, but alcohol was the thing that allowed me to switch off. Drinking soon became my crutch, and it got worse and worse. I had severe anxiety problems, so one of my doctors gave me a benzodiazepine and told me to take it as needed.

I was drinking and taking benzos—that led to a cataclysmic breakdown. Previously, drinking had been a subconscious coping mechanism, but this time it was a choice. I had made a conscious decision to get obliterated. I remember being in a couple of bars and drinking heavily. I don't remember the walk home, but I bought sleeping pills, blended them up and drank them. I must have called someone because I woke up having had my stomach pumped, and I was then on suicide watch in a psychiatric unit.

A doctor said, "You don't need more medication. You have a drinking problem; you need to stop." When I saw myself through that lens, I knew I had to get my shit together. It was the eureka moment.

When I gave up drinking, I was on my knees. Everything was foggy, and there was no focus or structure. Everyone said I should leave my job, too. I fundamentally disagreed with that, so instead I shifted my role from bartender to operations manager.

I threw myself into recovery and a bunch of things happened: I lost 40 lb and I became a lot more structured in my work–life balance. Now, I take that same focus into my relationships, so that I'm as present as I can be with my girlfriend. I work out a lot, I have two dogs, and I have plenty of things I enjoy doing outside of work.

I was ambitious with my sobriety. People know our bars and know me, so I put it out right away that I have these problems. I wanted to destigmatize it, to get more people involved in the conversation.

We're constantly barraged with messaging around alcohol, and it's at the center of most social activities. When anyone asks about changing their consumption, I always say, "You've gotta want it." It's not easy.

I'm fully behind inclusivity for people who do not drink or are moderating, and groups such as Club Soda are fundamental to that.

MY STORY:

MY MOOD

THIS SPACE IS FOR YOUR NOTES ON YOUR FEELINGS, EMOTIONAL WELL-BEING, AND YOUR ABILITY TO COPE WITH STRESS AND BOREDOM. ALSO JOT DOWN THINGS THAT YOU ARE AWARE OF AS WELL AS ANYTHING ELSE THAT IS HELPFUL TO YOU.

These notes pages work alongside the prompts across pages 92–103. Complete in the spaces below or copy into your journal or notebook.

FEELING GOOD

Explore what brings you pleasure day to day (see also pages 92–93). Think in terms of all the senses.

Touch

Taste

Smell

Hearing

Sight

OPENING THE BOX

Explore any strong feelings and what might make you sad (see also pages 94–95).

What makes me sad, stressed, or anxious?

How can I live well with these feelings?

GOING DEEPER WITH HALT

Tackle these big questions (see also pages 102–103) when you are feeling strong and emotionally supported.

Hunger: What am I hungry for in life?

Anger: What frustrations are holding me back?

Loneliness: What do I need to be happy in my own company?

Tiredness: How am I meeting my need for rest and self-care?

ANY OTHER NOTES

DRINKING AND OTHER PEOPLE

SOCIALIZING // CONFIDENCE // SUPPORT //
CELEBRATIONS // DATING // SEX //
RELATIONSHIPS // CHILDREN // WORK //
MELISSA'S STORY // MY STORY: MY RELATIONSHIPS

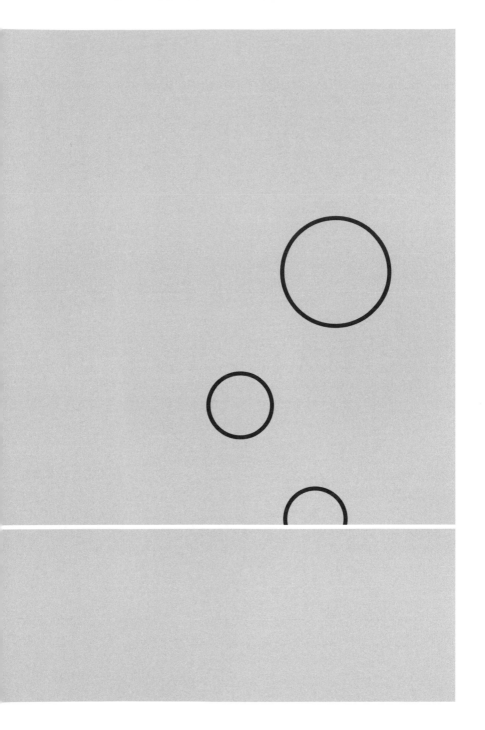

SOCIALIZING

Social connection and interaction are good for us. But as a mindful drinker, you might notice how much socializing centers on alcohol. Drinking pops up all over the place, and not just at parties and weddings. From book clubs to work conferences, we seem unable to get together with people without alcohol.

> **Whether you change your drinking by quitting or moderating, you can learn to socialize alcohol-free.**

DRINKING AND OTHER PEOPLE

If you are anxious, you might find that it gets worse around other people. Social anxiety might be a reason you drink more than you want to, just to cope with being with others. But like other types of anxiety-related drinking (see page 98), drinking just masks the problem. We may be spending time with other people, but are we really feeling a connection with them? Not so much.

Increasing numbers of us live alone, and we're more likely to drink more in private, too. So getting out and building a social life that doesn't center on alcohol can be an important part of combatting the loneliness that can be a trigger for our drinking (see HALT, page 102).

SOCIALIZING ALCOHOL-FREE

Even if you are moderating, there will be days on which you don't drink alcohol. But your social life and plans don't need to change as a result. However you change your drinking, it's useful to learn to socialize alcohol-free.

If you tended to drink with other people, don't isolate yourself now. Remember, being with other people is fundamentally good for you. Socializing does not have to mean partying hard; you can have an active social life without a hangover the next day.

If you are going out with friends, make some if–then plans (see page 57) and practice ways of saying "no." But remember that if someone offers to buy you a drink, it's because they want to include you socially. You can politely ask for a soft drink. If you don't entirely trust them not to order a measure of gin with your tonic, offer to help them at the bar.

You might not want to socialize with your old posse of drinking buddies, but making new friends doesn't have to be difficult. Join meet-up groups, become a volunteer, or take an evening class. Get to know people in environments that don't center on drinking. You can find other people who enjoy the things you do. From cosplay conventions to walking groups, many Club Soda members have built amazing, alcohol-free social lives.

The quality of friendship matters much more than the quantity of acquaintances. Better one good friend than a party of strangers.

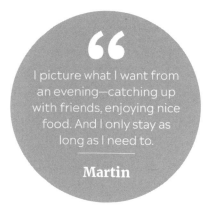

> **"**
> I picture what I want from
> an evening—catching up
> with friends, enjoying nice
> food. And I only stay as
> long as I need to.
>
> **Martin**

CONFIDENCE

If we feel awkward around other people, particularly in unfamiliar social settings, we can find ourselves relying on liquid courage. Alcohol relaxes our inhibitions so it works—at first. Before long, the drinking catches up with us. Feeling friendly and outgoing after one drink can turn into being a mess after too many. Dutch courage is impossible to control.

As you change your drinking, you may need to discover how to be confident around other people without alcohol. Trust us when we say: you can do this. You can learn to unlock the confidence you already have.

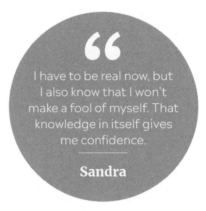

> 66
> I have to be real now, but I also know that I won't make a fool of myself. That knowledge in itself gives me confidence.
>
> **Sandra**

WHAT DOES CONFIDENCE LOOK LIKE?

You walk into a crowded room. All eyes turn to you. You smile. You approach the most important person in the room and engage them in sparkling conversation. If this is your mental image of what social confidence looks like, you might be setting yourself up to fail. In reality, confidence comes in much smaller packages.

Your first steps to confidence in social settings might seem small to others, but they can be big for you:

- smiling at a stranger
- sitting in a coffee shop by yourself
- asking someone about their day

Confidence isn't about making yourself the center of attention. Confidence is about being comfortable in your own skin.

FORGETTING YOURSELF

Ironically, one of the ways you can become more confident is by not trying to be confident at all. Forgetting yourself is something that alcohol helped you with; it numbed your feelings of discomfort in social situations. You became more confident because you stopped thinking about yourself.

You can still do this, but without the drink. Confidence grows with practice. Below are some ideas to feel more confident in any social setting:

Ask other people about themselves to shift the focus away from you. Build a repertoire of questions.

Listen carefully and follow people's interests. "Tell me more about ..." is a great way to get over a quiet patch.

Politely move on if a conversation isn't working out. Sometimes, discussions just run their course, so don't be embarrassed about excusing yourself.

Have a nonalcoholic drink. Even a glass of sparkling mineral water gives you something to do with your hands, and you'll feel less like you stand out.

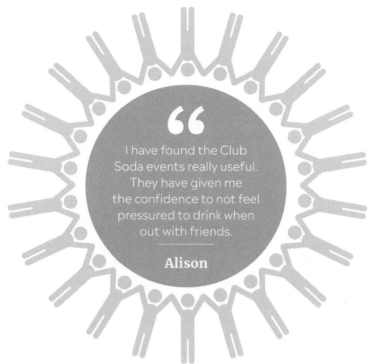

"

I have found the Club Soda events really useful. They have given me the confidence to not feel pressured to drink when out with friends.

Alison

SUPPORT

Socializing gives us a chance to meet like-minded people who can support us as we change our drinking. Social connection is one of the reasons we started Club Soda. None of us should have to change our drinking alone. But finding places to hang out together can be tricky. Support groups in dusty church halls can be helpful, but they're hardly fun. Ultimately, what's important is having a group of people around you who support your decisions and are there for you when you need them.

That's why Club Soda actively works with pubs, bars, and restaurants to help them improve their range of no- and low-alcohol drinks, so we can create a world where nobody feels out of place if they're not drinking.

Club Soda members organize social events, lunches, and evening drinks to meet new people and see old friends. All our events are alcohol-free because, even if you are moderating, it's good to have an opportunity to socialize without drinking. Now you're part of Club Soda, you can come along or organize an event of your own—head to joinclubsoda.com to find out more.

DIFFICULT PEOPLE

Spending time with other people who are also changing their drinking can be all the support we need. But it's unrealistic to expect that everyone who currently features in your life will be supportive. Especially in social contexts centered on drinking, not drinking upsets social norms.

You don't even need to talk about changing your drinking—some people will react if they see you without a glass of wine or bottle of beer. Your decisions can be surprisingly unsettling for others. Although many people will react with curiosity, some may become defensive about their own drinking; they might deal with their discomfort by trying to get you to have an alcoholic drink. This can be distressing. It's key to understand a few things:

- **If you drink, it won't actually make them feel better**—and it's really about you, not them.
- **You can say "no,"** though you might have to be a broken record for a while to get the point across.
- **You can't expect them to be enthusiastic about your choices**, but you do deserve respect.
- **You don't have to tackle the issue right now**—if they are too drunk to reason with, now is not the time to sort things out.

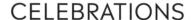

CELEBRATIONS

Your first party or wedding as a mindful drinker is an important milestone. Before you changed your drinking, you would probably have accepted invitations without a second thought. Even if you knew a hangover would come your way, you threw yourself in. Now, though, it may feel a little daunting.

Celebrations require a little thought and advanced planning. And once you're there, all the skills you've learned in socializing (see page 112), confidence (see page 114), and dealing with difficult people (see page 117) will come into play. This is your moment to shine.

PARTIES

Partying as a mindful drinker is actually one of the easier things you might do socially. If parties in your social circle tend to be "bring your own bottle" affairs, take something delicious for yourself to drink.

Remember that you never have to stay at a party for a moment longer than you want to. If you're no longer enjoying the vibe, it's OK to go home. In fact, you might want to say goodbye to your host the moment you see them, just in case you don't get a chance to chat later. You can then make an embarrassment-free exit if you need to.

Our only word of caution about parties is that you might need to hide the bottle you bring with you! As the booze runs low, and other guests look for any mixer to go with the terrible spirit they find at the back of the liquor cabinet, your carefully chosen drink could disappear into their glasses.

WEDDINGS

You only need to glance at wedding stationery to see how closely we associate celebrations and champagne. Attending a catered event requires some thought if you are not going to be left sharing the children's orange juice.

Be clear with whoever has invited you that you don't want to drink alcohol at their event. This should be no more controversial than saying you are a vegetarian or require a gluten-free meal. Any good caterer should be able to accommodate your wishes for nonalcoholic beverages.

Options might still be limited, but ask for what you want. Depending on how well you know the person who issued the invitation, you might wish to have a chat about the options that will be available. Bear in mind that they might not have considered the issue before you mention it.

Our guide to no- and low-alcohol drinks later in this book is a useful place to start the conversation (see page 138).

DATING

For many of us, dating and drinking go hand in hand. Meeting for a drink is the default option. However, you are changing your drinking, so you don't have to follow this social norm. Especially if you are moderating, it can be eye-opening to experience what dating alcohol-free is like. It is different—and it requires some extra creativity and planning.

FINDING A DATE

Many of us introduce ourselves to the world with a glass of something in our hand. Whether it's a colorful cocktail or a tumbler of whiskey, our profile pictures on dating sites and social media can be incredibly alcohol-centric. Now is perhaps the time to review your profile image. Do your profile pictures show the world who you were or who you are becoming?

TELLING YOUR DATE

Many of us get anxious about telling a potential date that we don't drink often, much, or at all. On photo-based dating and hook-up apps it can be less

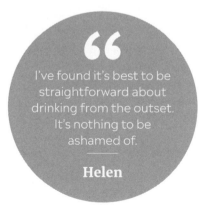

> **"**
> I've found it's best to be straightforward about drinking from the outset. It's nothing to be ashamed of.
>
> ---
>
> **Helen**

of an issue. If you write a dating profile, you could say something about drinking, or you could decide to tell your date in person. Whatever you choose, you don't need to justify yourself to anyone. Although being a mindful drinker may be a big deal for you, it's simply another fact about you for anyone else.

When you talk about drinking, some potential dates may react badly. But it means you get to weed out those who don't support your choices early on.

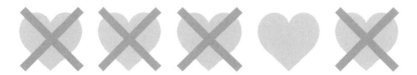

GOING ON A DATE

Once you've snagged your hot date, take the initiative. You can avoid drinking by doing what you want to do. Dates don't have to be in the evening, for instance, nor do they have to be three hours long or involve alcohol at all. Lunch, coffee, a museum, walking, a farmer's market, roller skating, rock climbing ... the options are as limitless as your imagination.

LONG-TERM DATING

If you find it difficult to deal with your date's drinking, you don't have to see them again. Even if they are otherwise perfect, it's not your job to "save" them. That said, the opposite also holds true—don't date people just because they are alcohol-free. There are other things that are important to you, so make sure they tick all your boxes, not just the drinking one.

A date that doesn't revolve around drinking gives you a chance to get to know someone better and you can present yourself exactly as you are. If you decide to take things further, a clear-headed assessment of your compatibility is a good way to start any long-term relationship (see page 124).

SEX

Alcohol-free sex can be daunting. Without a drink inside them, some people find themselves confronted by an awkwardness in their naked bodies. Others might be embarrassed when talking openly about desires, and even unsure whether they enjoy such physical intimacy at all. But the fact is, drinking too much can stop us from becoming aroused and can make it harder to climax.

Whether you are quitting or moderating, alcohol-free sex can be one of the best things about being a mindful drinker—at any time, day or night.

GET COMFORTABLE

If the need to drink has got wrapped up in your sex life because you feel awkward naked, spending time alone naked can help. Explore the pleasures of your own body with all your senses. Learn to love your own body and what it can do, just as it is.

As you get comfortable in your skin, the kind of sex you want to have might change. Talking about sex might take some courage if you've been relying on alcohol to overcome your embarrassment. Be honest about your

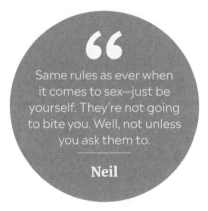

> Same rules as ever when it comes to sex—just be yourself. They're not going to bite you. Well, not unless you ask them to.
>
> **Neil**

desires, how you feel, and what you want. And remember, in the heat of the moment, the best consent is enthusiastic and vocal.

BE FULLY PRESENT

You're more likely to have the sex you want to have if you are alcohol-free. You can be fully conscious in your own body, and experience all the unfiltered sensations and pleasures of physical intimacy. You can be fully present for someone else, too, and attentive to their needs and desires.

Being alcohol-free makes it easier to talk about and to use condoms and other protection against sexually transmitted infections, so you're more likely to have safer sex. If you have the kind of sex that could lead to pregnancy, it's important to know that your fertility will improve as you change your drinking, so you might want to rethink your choice of contraception.

Alcohol-free leads to better pillow-talk, as you're less likely to crash into a drunken slumber the moment you finish. Enjoy this moment of connection.

Alcohol and sexual assault

Drinking is involved in at least half of all cases of sexual assault. But it's not just that alcohol makes clear conversations about consent more difficult. It's also that drinking can both provoke aggression and leave us vulnerable, unable to protect ourselves.

Sexual assault—in fact, any kind of unwanted sexual behavior—is never your fault, even if you have been drinking. If you are too drunk to give consent, you deserve to be cared for, not blamed or shamed.

If you have been sexually assaulted, seek the support you need. You can find helpful organizations in the resources section (see page 208).

RELATIONSHIPS

Change can put any relationship—even the happiest ones—under stress. Every relationship has a different degree of tolerance for change. Some of us actively expect our partners to grow over the course of our lives together, while others want our partners to stay exactly as they are.

In an ideal world, our partners would be our most enthusiastic cheerleaders, encouraging us to become who we are. Meanwhile, back in the real world, we know that isn't always the case.

Relationships unfold each day in the things that we think and feel, in the words that we say and in the things that we do. So, if drinking together has been a big part of what you do in your relationships, pay attention to what happens next.

TALKING TO YOUR PARTNER

You know best how to approach conversations with your partner.

- **Be honest and brave**. Remember that whatever you say is about you, and not about them. You can't change them, any more than they could have changed you. You've decided to do this for yourself. You'd love their support, but you're not asking them to change for you.

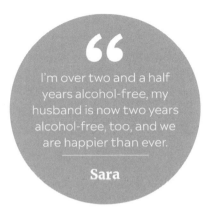

> **"**
> I'm over two and a half years alcohol-free, my husband is now two years alcohol-free, too, and we are happier than ever.
>
> **Sara**

- **Be clear about your intentions, make good plans, and keep track** of how things are going. Make sure you have a fridge stocked with alternatives you know you'll enjoy, especially if you used to drink at home with your partner. You can still spend time together, even if your drinks are different.

LIVING WITH SOMEONE WHO DRINKS

We won't sugarcoat this pill. Living with someone who drinks more than is good for them, and who doesn't want to change, can be hard. As you change, you might struggle with such a partner's drinking. But even if it all feels like a mess, you can work it out. Remember that they might have had problems dealing with your drinking in the past, too. You may want support to help you talk to each other (see page 208). Finding kindness, patience, and tolerance for your partner can be emotionally draining, especially when you are going through a period of change. So remember to be kind to yourself.

Whatever else you do, reach out to others. You are not alone. There are many Club Soda members who have been exactly where you are, and who have tackled their relationship issues in different ways. Find people who will listen without judgement, and who will help you discover what works for you.

CHILDREN

Lots of us have happy memories of childhood, but sadly that's not a universal experience. Some of us feel lucky to have escaped our childhoods relatively unscathed, and are bruised and battered by them. Whatever your childhood was like, growing up can be a real test of human resilience.

Tragically, some parents take their children's ability to bounce back for granted, treating their well-being with casual disregard. But many parents worry. We worry that we have passed on our worst habits to our kids. Worse, we worry that we have damaged them beyond repair.

The skills you have already learned as a mindful drinker can help you with your children. You can pay attention to your children and act with intention toward them. It takes conscious effort to change your approach to parenting, but it is possible to make a difference.

YOUNG CHILDREN

However young your children are, you can be certain that they notice your behavior when you are drinking more than you want to. But let go of your guilt. How you act now as a mindful drinker will have an impact. Your children will begin to respond positively as you become more present, less volatile, and better able to respond to their needs.

If you are home with young children for much of the day, stress can be a challenge, to say the least. Making time to care for yourself

> 66
> I'm more fun, more energetic, less stressed in the mornings. I'm not a perfect parent now, but I know I'm a nicer mommy.
>
> **Judy**

can feel impossible, but even just 60 seconds spent with your eyes closed, focusing on your breathing, can help you feel calmer.

Remember if–then plans (see page 57)? These can be so helpful when you are dealing with day-to-day parenting. If you know that there are predictable points in your day when reaching for a bottle seems like the only thing to do, it can be useful to start some new habits to support you (see page 172).

TEENAGERS

Take it as a given that your teenager will experiment with drinking and that they may try to hide this from you. Your parenting skills might be exemplary, but at some point, you will be told you know nothing about modern teens. You'll be branded a hypocrite and a bedroom door will be slammed in your face.

You can help them, though. Your honesty about your own experiences can be powerful. Talking to teenagers about drinking can be embarrassing and uncomfortable, but be assured that—at some level—they do listen.

As they get older, they might want to drink alcohol at home. Much like living with a partner who drinks (see page 125), if you are alcohol-free and feel safest if you don't have alcohol at home, this can be difficult to deal with. It can be tempting to hide behind rules and prohibitions as a way of dealing with your own discomfort, but it's probably more helpful—to you and your teenagers—to have an honest conversation about what's going on. If you let your teenagers understand the challenges you are dealing with, you might be surprised by their capacity for empathy.

Don't be afraid to apologize and admit when you get things wrong. For your kids, learning to accept you as an imperfect human being and loving you anyway is a vital part of growing up.

WORK

Working and drinking can be closely entwined. Some professions have a reputation for it, such as the financial sector, the hospitality industry, and advertising. But other professionals, such as nurses, teachers, and lawyers, are quietly drinking more than they should without the rest of us noticing.

Unless we work entirely alone, it's likely that alcohol will show up at some point in our working life. In many companies, after-work drinks are the norm, and seen as a crucial moment for colleagues to unwind together and to bond. Many of us have stories to tell about office parties that got out of control, but social events with coworkers can be a big part of what makes work enjoyable.

Away from our workplaces, conferences often end with cocktail receptions, and evening networking events often revolve around wine. And then comes client entertainment. Would anyone seriously take a prospective client out to dinner and only offer them water?

How can we live in a work-hard, play-hard culture as mindful drinkers?

PLANNING AHEAD

As with any other situation, having clear intentions and a robust plan will help you (see pages 48 and 52). Remember, even if the person offering you a drink is your boss, drinking alcohol is not compulsory. You can say "no" and still be active in the social life of your workplace. Your ability to get through a work event without drinking might be just the encouragement that someone else needs to join in, when before they might have gone home early.

Not drinking is becoming increasingly common. As a mindful drinker, you'll notice all the other people who don't drink often, much, or at all— pregnant colleagues, people who drive home from work, and coworkers who abstain for religious reasons. There is always safety in numbers, and it's never a bad thing to build new connections in a workplace.

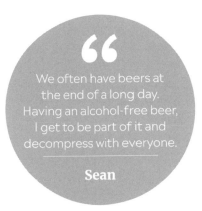

> **66**
> We often have beers at
> the end of a long day.
> Having an alcohol-free beer,
> I get to be part of it and
> decompress with everyone.
>
> **Sean**

That said, some social events can be avoided fairly easily. But if drinking is harder to miss, say at a work conference, find out as much as you can in advance about the venue and catering arrangements. A good caterer wouldn't dream of feeding meat to vegetarians. Likewise, there's no good reason for them to ignore the needs of those not drinking alcohol. Be proactive and ask for what you want.

GETTING SUPPORT

At times of stress in our personal lives, work can feel like a refuge. You might not feel comfortable talking to colleagues about your home life, and that is OK. Work in itself can be a useful distraction.

Many employers have programs to support the health and well-being of their staff. You might be able to access confidential information and advice through such programs. In many cases, the issues you raise don't even have to be work-related. If you are dealing with difficult issues in your life—whether or not they are related to changing your drinking—your employer may have a program that could help you.

HOW I CHANGED MY DRINKING: **MELISSA'S STORY**

I was 13 when I first drank. I woke up in the hospital having had my stomach pumped. That was just the beginning of an unhealthy love affair with drink. I gravitated toward the party crowd, seeking attention through wild drinking. That continued through high school into adulthood. I was a heavy drinker, and I'd black out a lot, too. But I wanted everyone to think, "Wow, Melissa is a fun party girl!"

I married an awesome guy, and we have two 17-year-olds now. I used to think to myself, "I'm a successful realtor, I'm a great mom, and life is in a beautiful place." I also thought that drinking didn't control my life, but I was blacking out about six times a year. That wasn't ok. Blackouts represent a huge trauma in my past, and it's hard waking up and dealing with those memories.

I've done "dry January" every year since turning 21. It helped, breaking the cycle every year. But it also tricked me into thinking "I'm fine, everything's under control." I realized nothing changes in those time-outs unless I do the work on what's behind my drinking.

I'm not drinking at the moment and I'm asking myself questions. What is it about going out with my friends that makes me nervous?

What makes it hard to look at the waiter and say "No thanks, I just want a club soda"? Why does that feel shameful?

I don't want to set a bad example for my children. It matters what they see, that they know that there needs to be careful thought around drink. I'm extremely candid, open, and honest with them because I think that it's important to be. And I think because I've been that way, they've grown up making some really good decisions. They're not partyers. They run around with a pretty solid group of friends. They have tried alcohol and we've talked about it.

My husband and I have just got back from a vacation in Mexico. Normally we'd drink cocktails and beers, it's part of our routine. I kept thinking about how we can get away and not make alcohol part of it. I asked, "What does drinking give me, and what does it take away?"

So, this time I set intentions. I got up every morning and headed for a jog on the beach. I finished one book and started another. I took kombuchas and shrubs out with me. I gave myself the opportunity for meaningful successes. Usually, I come home and need a vacation from the vacation, but this time I came home feeling replenished.

MY STORY:

MY RELATIONSHIPS

THIS SPACE IS FOR YOUR NOTES. THIS
SECTION LOOKS AT SOCIALIZING,
SUPPORT, YOUR FAMILY AND FRIENDS,
AND WORK. JOT DOWN THINGS THAT
YOU BECOME AWARE OF AS WELL AS
ANYTHING ELSE THAT IS HELPFUL TO YOU.

These notes pages work alongside the prompts across pages 112–129.
Complete in the spaces below or copy into your journal or notebook.

MY SOCIAL LIFE

Explore this section (see also pages 112–119) to identify what could help you
keep up with friends and family without alcohol being at the center.

What have I noticed about alcohol's role in my social life?

What social events are coming up? What plans will I make so that I can enjoy them without drinking?

What support do I want or need from others?

MY PERSONAL RELATIONSHIPS

Explore all aspects of your relationships (see also pages 120–129) to identify what would be helpful to make these work alcohol-free.

How is my **love life** changing?

How is my **sex life** changing?

How are **my relationships** generally changing?

How is my relationship with **my family** changing?

How is my relationship with **my friends** changing?

How is my **work life** changing?

ANY OTHER NOTES

The final part of this book is full of useful advice to support you to live as a mindful drinker.

You'll find a guide to choosing alcohol-free drinks—from beers, wines, and spirits to tonics, shrubs, and home brews—so you can find something exciting to put in your mouth. There's a chapter of advanced behavior change techniques to supercharge your mindful drinking skills. And, in case you run into difficulties, you'll find information on some of the most common problems you might face after you change your drinking and what to do about them.

Remember, being a mindful drinker isn't a solo endurance sport. There are thousands of people just like you. So turn to the end of the book for information on how to find the others (see page 206).

PART 3
LIVING

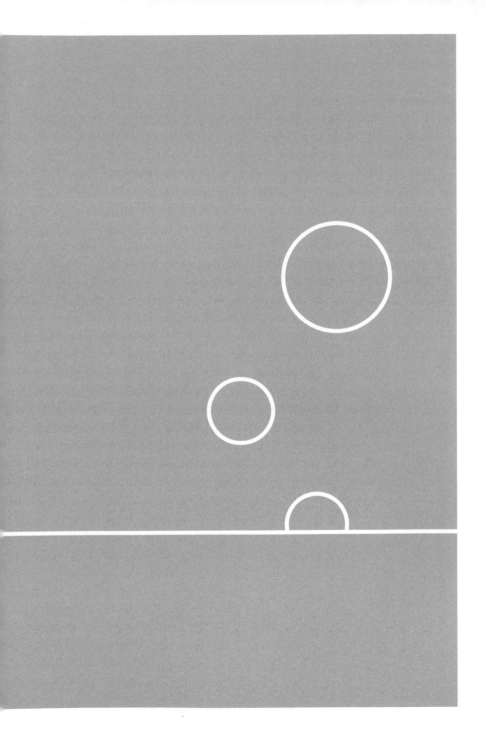

WHAT TO
DRINK INSTEAD

CHOICES, CHOICES // 0.5% IS ALCOHOL-FREE //
WHAT TO ORDER // BEERS // WINES //
SPIRITS // TONICS AND MIXERS // SODAS //
SHRUBS // HOME BREWS // JUSSI'S STORY //
MY STORY: WHAT I'M DRINKING

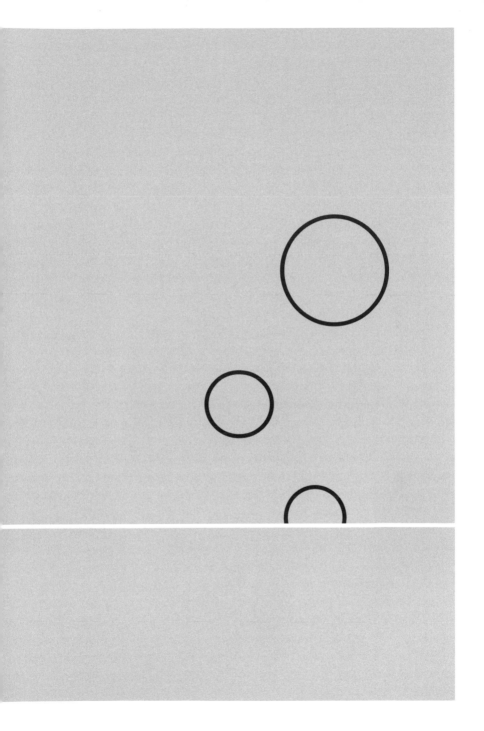

CHOICES, CHOICES

What do mindful drinkers drink instead of alcohol?

This is one of the most common questions we hear in Club Soda. Many of us find ourselves frustrated by a limited choice of high-sugar options, such as cola or orange juice, and few of us are satisfied with water (even fizzy water) alone. We want more, and rightly so.

Happily, there are lots of alcohol-free drinks to satisfy an adult palate. This chapter will help you find new products to try, from alcohol-free alternatives to adult soft drinks. We're not recommending specific drinks here—there are far too many to choose from—but check in with us online to get our regular drink reviews.

Reduced- or low-alcohol drinks can be super-useful if you are moderating, but there are too many to mention. So here we focus on alcohol-free drinks— though what we mean by alcohol-free might surprise you (see page 142).

YOUR NEW FAVORITE DRINK

You've probably had your favorite tipple for years. Whether it's beer, wine, or gin, an alternative for your mindful drinking future exists.

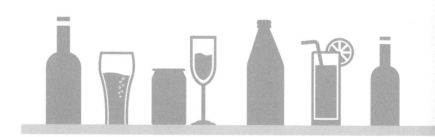

Think about your favorite alcoholic drinks and what you enjoyed about those. Taste will have played a starring role, so you probably weren't consuming them solely for their alcoholic content. Consider the flavor profiles that you enjoy. Maybe botanicals get you going, or perhaps you enjoy fruity characters? There is nothing to say that you cannot continue to enjoy these kinds of flavors now that you are drinking mindfully.

Consider the habits that surrounded your drinking, too. When finding alternatives, you are looking not only to replace a drink, but also to replace the sense of occasion that came with it. Perhaps you associate a glass of red wine in the evening with unwinding and letting go of the day. It is important to remember that unwinding is still yours to indulge in. Find an alternative that you still consider to be an evening drink for slow sipping.

You may find that as you change your drinking, you become more sensitive to sweet flavors. This may alter your enjoyment of certain drinks. Notice this and seek out new things that you prefer. Your taste buds might change completely, so keep searching for things you love.

You deserve to take pleasure in the drinks you consume. Use your mindful drinking skills—paying attention and acting with intention—and choose drinks that are best for you.

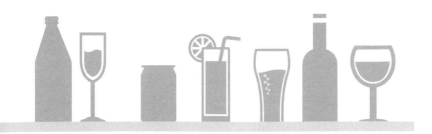

0.5% IS ALCOHOL-FREE

One of the most frequently asked questions in Club Soda is about drinks that contain 0.5% alcohol. These drinks can be confusing and worrying, particularly for people who are going alcohol-free. Some drinks are labeled as alcohol-free, while others aren't—and a few drinks even say they are alcohol-free and not alcohol-free on the same label! People who don't drink alcohol for religious reasons can worry that 0.5% alcohol is still alcohol and should be avoided. And then Club Soda comes along, actively promoting 0.5% alcohol beer at our Mindful Drinking Festivals.

How is anyone supposed to make any sense of it? What does 0.5% mean?

99.5% water and other ingredients

0.5% alcohol

Saying that a drink contains 0.5% alcohol by volume means that it is 99.5% water and other nonalcoholic ingredients. Labeling regulations are complex and vary in different countries, but in many parts of the world 0.5% drinks are labeled as alcohol-free.

Drinks containing up to 0.5% cannot cause intoxication and are completely safe for drivers and those who are pregnant. That's because the amount of alcohol contained in these drinks is negligible—your body can safely process this tiny amount before it has any effect on you.

DON'T WORRY ABOUT 0.5%

Some people worry about 0.5%, so it can help to understand what it really means. You'll need to make up your own mind on whether these drinks are right for you. Read on to get a fuller picture.

In reality, 0.5% is a *trace* of alcohol. Fermentation is a natural process and one that we associate with alcoholic drinks. But it is also part of the production of many foods, especially fermented foods. We don't tend to worry about the amounts of alcohol in food, because to eat enough to become intoxicated would be impossible. In fact, many people aren't even aware that there is alcohol in food products from rye bread to soy sauce. So why worry about drinks?

You'd never guess but many drinks—ripe banana smoothies, for instance—can contain greater amounts of alcohol than alcohol-free beers, wines, and spirits. What's good to know is that 0.5% drinks often contain considerably fewer calories than sugary alternatives. Alcohol-free beer is even lauded for its isotonic properties. And, of course, all 0.5% drinks can be helpful in changing your drinking—and they are great in their own right.

USING 0.5% TO SUSTAIN MINDFUL DRINKING

Even though you can't become physically dependent on 0.5% alternatives, how you feel about what you drink still matters. The experience of the flavor and consistency of an alcohol-free drink might trigger a desire for its full-strength counterpart. If you have gone alcohol-free, this might be a problem.

But drinks of up to 0.5% can support you to change your drinking. You'll find them in bars, pubs, and restaurants, too, so they can help you build and sustain your mindful drinking social life.

Ultimately, the only way to know what works for you is to experiment and to pay attention to what happens. It is completely up to you to decide whether or not 0.5% is right for you.

> 66
>
> I wouldn't have changed my drinking without 0.5% beer. It's my new normal. I'd choose it over alcoholic beer any time.
>
> **Dru**

WHAT TO ORDER

While there are new products coming to market all the time, many bars, restaurants, and social spaces still don't present a good enough range for those of us who are not drinking.

Going to the bar and ordering can be daunting if we want something delicious and nonalcoholic. It's no surprise that many people feel anxious when trying to get what they want. To compound this, many venues will hide their alcohol-free beers and similar drinks in the bottom of the fridge or in unlit corners, so it isn't always clear what they have to offer.

To make the whole process simpler, and less worrisome, look for venues that list alcohol-free options on their menu, especially those with menus on their website that you can check before you visit. This means you can plan ahead and feel more confident when ordering.

ORDERING "OFF MENU"

If you discover the options are limited, bitters are a good way to add a mature twist to soda water or a soft drink. Ask the bartender to pop a few drops in a ginger beer or sparkling water to see how their flavor makes a big difference. Although bitters do contain alcohol, once diluted their effect is negligible.

And if all else fails, sneak in your own favorite cordial to jazz up tonic water. Elderflower is always a winner.

> Tell the bartender that you aren't drinking alcohol and you're looking for a really interesting drink. They should be ready to help you find something.

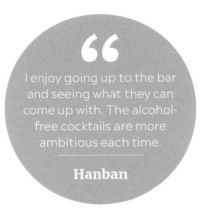

> **"** I enjoy going up to the bar and seeing what they can come up with. The alcohol-free cocktails are more ambitious each time.
>
> **Hanban**

Don't forget, you are just as important as any other drinking customer. If you found the options to be lacking, give constructive feedback. You can politely suggest the manager look into alternatives or leave an online review if you aren't comfortable discussing it in person. This will help change the drinks landscape and encourage venues to improve their offering. Sadly, many bar managers overlook the needs of people who aren't drinking alcohol, so try to gently open their eyes. Venues are missing an opportunity to increase their income. "I'd have spent more if you stocked *insert preferred drink here* in the fridge" will always get their attention!

THINK VALUE FOR MONEY, NOT PRICE

Many of the most interesting no- and low-alcohol drinks will be priced similarly to their full-strength counterparts. This is because the raw materials and labor costs involved in production are often the same, and sometimes higher if there have been extra processes to remove alcohol.

So try to shift your mind-set from the idea that alcohol drives price. Think instead of how something has been crafted to satisfy your need for flavor, and let this guide you in your perception of value for money.

BEER

If you are looking for an alcohol-free beer, you are in luck. From uncomplicated lagers to complex ales, huge numbers of alcohol-free beers are emerging onto the market, from international beer brands and small craft brewers alike.

If you tend to drink straightforward lagers, this is all you need to know: many big beer brands are investing significant time and money to create alcohol-free beers, and most of them are great. Enjoy them ice cold.

But you need more information if you are a craft beer fan. To understand how to choose a good alcohol-free beer, it helps to understand a little about how it is made.

HOW THEY MAKE ALCOHOL-FREE BEER

Beer is made from four simple ingredients: malt, water, yeast, and hops. Malt is steeped in hot water, to break the grain down and release its sugars. This creates a hot sweet liquid called wort, which is cooled before yeast is added. The yeast consumes the sugars, leaving carbon dioxide and alcohol behind. The hops then add flavor, bitterness, and aroma.

So how do brewers make beer that's alcohol-free? There are basically two ways. The first method is to make beer as usual and then remove the alcohol. But it's hard to do this without changing the flavor. The cheapest and quickest way is to heat the beer, so the alcohol boils off. This is simple, but it leaves a disappointing taste behind. A slightly better approach involves a similar process but under pressure. The gold standard for alcohol removal, though, is a process known as reverse osmosis, but this requires brewers to make a significant investment in the technology needed. The resulting beer, however, is identical to its full-strength equivalent, just without the alcohol.

The second way, which some craft brewers favor, is to brew the beer to the strength required, by using lazy yeasts (strains of yeast that stop working quickly and so don't produce much alcohol), or by halting the fermentation process. This method generally results in a better-tasting drink, which overcomes some of the classic complaints about alcohol-free beer—that it is thin, sweet, and lacking complexity.

TOP TIPS FOR NO- OR LOW-ALCOHOL BEER

- **Hunt down small producers and microbreweries**. There are some that only produce alcohol free beer. They are often passionate about their craft and would love to tell you about what they do.
- **Be careful about storing beer in clear or green bottles**. These are at risk of becoming what's known as "light-struck," meaning that UV rays affect the flavor, giving rise to skunky aromas. Stick to beer in brown bottles or cans or keep it somewhere dark and cool.
- **Try new things**. Look for wheat beers for a fuller body and stouts for rich, roasted flavors. Some online retailers sell mixed boxes of alcohol-free beers, so you can find something that you love.
- **Look out for "small beer"** if you are moderating. This medieval-style beer is 2.8% or less and can be a good way of pacing yourself, especially alternated with an alcohol-free beer.

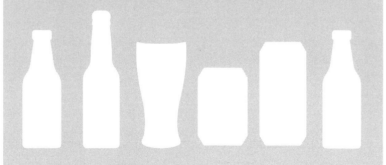

WINE

Wine is such an expansive category that it is hard to generalize, but we'll try. Broadly speaking, alcohol-free white and sparkling wines are better than alcohol-free red wines. This is not to say that producers aren't working hard to improve this. Creating a good-quality, alcohol-free wine is a challenge the drinks industry is slowly rising to.

HOW THEY MAKE ALCOHOL-FREE WINE

Wine making takes time. Vineyards not only make wine, but they also grow the grapes used to make it. A great amount of time is spent maintaining the land and tending the vines. When harvest time comes, grapes are gathered and winemakers set about turning them into wine. This means that they have only one chance each year to produce the best possible wine, and they have to then set about de-alcoholizing it.

Wine is even more sensitive to heat than beer (see page 146), easily becoming oxidized or caramelized. So, many winemakers invest in expensive centrifuges and filtration systems to remove the alcohol from their wines.

Whereas brewers can taste their product along the way and add more ingredients to improve its flavor, winemakers cannot. Wine is a simple fermentation of grapes that relies heavily on its alcohol content to bring viscosity and body to the drink. Once you strip out the alcohol, you are left with something that does not coat the palate as a full-strength wine would.

Alcohol-free wine tends to lack complexity, particularly if heat has been involved in the process of removing the alcohol. You'll find that red wine does maintain a strong tannic character but often lacks rich flavor to support this. So you may find things are a little imbalanced on the tongue.

While you're exploring the world of alcohol-free wines, check out the top tips we've gathered from our years of research (see opposite).

TOP TIPS FOR WHITE AND SPARKLING WINE

- **Shell out for quality.** Price matters when choosing alcohol-free wine. Cheap blends of grapes make poor-quality wines. Single-grape varieties tend to make a better-quality product.
- **Serve well chilled.** Because complex flavors aren't always top of the agenda for white and sparkling wines, you can and should enjoy them cold.
- **Consider mixers.** Add some soda to transform alcohol-free white wine into a great spritzer or create a champagne-style cocktail with extra fruit, cordial, or bitters to a base of alcohol-free sparkling wine.

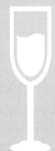

TOP TIPS FOR RED WINE

- **Keep trying new ones**. Red wine can be trickier to replace. But some producers are experimenting with adding botanicals to de-alcoholized red wine to replicate the complexity of flavor.
- **Choose an alcohol-free gluhwein** for an excellent seasonal party option with plenty of cloves, cinnamon, and citrus.
- **Consider switching to an alcohol-free craft beer**. The complexity of flavor can easily match that of a good red wine.
- **Add a splash of vinegar** to counter the sweetness and balance out the flavor of an alcohol-free red wine.

SPIRITS

Alcoholic spirits are enjoyed in a number of ways: neat, with mixers, or in cocktails. A whole array of flavors is displayed across the breadth of spirits available, from smoke, wood, and molasses to aniseed, vanilla, and juniper.

Spirits have an undeniable viscosity, and as they are much stronger than beer and wine, they have a far greater alcoholic burn. While flavor can be successfully recreated, the mouthfeel and heat of spirits are by far the hardest characteristics to replicate in alcohol-free versions.

Some alcohol-free spirits call themselves gin, rum, or something similar, but you'll notice that some brands remove themselves from preexisting categories, opting instead to describe themselves as botanicals or elixirs.

HOW THEY MAKE ALCOHOL-FREE SPIRITS

Much in the same way as beer (see page 146) or wine (see page 148), some of these products will be made to full strength, and the alcohol will then be stripped out. Alternatively, some will be made to replicate the flavors you might expect, but will never actually create any alcohol.

At present, botanical-based spirits are a little closer in flavor to their full-strength counterparts than dark spirits (such as whiskey and rum), but recreating the burn of alcohol remains a challenge.

Some producers are currently using capsaicin—extracted from the shells of chile seeds—to provide the warmth you feel at the back of the throat with alcoholic spirits. You may welcome this sensation, but beware of these drinks if you are sensitive to peppers!

TOP TIPS FOR ALCOHOL-FREE SPIRITS

- **Opt for quality and excellent flavor profiles**. Alcohol-free spirits can cost as much as their full-strength versions. Remember that you are paying for the excellent flavor, not the alcohol.

- **Mix up some cocktails**. You can use alcohol-free spirits to great effect in cocktails, but you may find you want to adjust quantities depending on the recipe. Juices and egg whites (often used in sours) can do a lot to bring texture and body to your drink.

- **Discover cocktail bitters** as these can bring extra layers of flavor when building a mixed drink. They can really aid in creating grown-up flavors for a fraction of the price of some alcohol-free spirits.

- **Try using syrups and cordials** to replicate the flavors you might find in rum such as vanilla and molasses.

- **Be creative when mixing your drinks**, and don't forget about the importance of "the serve" (see page 152). A beautiful glass, ice, and a garnish make a big difference to the drinking experience.

- **Consider whether you actually want to replace the alcohol at all.** For example, in a gin and tonic, it is often the taste of quinine (from the tonic) we enjoy, as well as the garnish and the ice clinking in the glass.

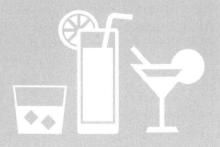

TONIC AND MIXERS

Tonics are a brilliant choice if you're looking for something low in calories and sugar and a little more grown-up in flavor. Many people overlook the importance of tonic when mixing with gin, assuming the flavor of the spirit is the most important thing, but tonic can be incredibly varied and it deserves credit as a stand-alone drink. Avoid the generic supermarket Indian tonic water stuff. You deserve more than quinine and fizz. Tonics now come with added citrus, herbal, spicy, or floral characters, so keep your eye out for interesting varieties to try.

As you change your drinking and your taste buds adjust accordingly, some of the mixers you would have enjoyed before may now seem too sweet. Look for small producers who are likely to use unusual ingredients to create more complex flavors rather than relying on sweetness. If you enjoyed lemonade before, consider looking for traditional or cloudy varieties that are likely to lean more toward bright, citric acidity than sugar. Seek out colas and sodas that focus on natural ingredients—they'll contain fewer sweeteners and additives and will have a much more authentic flavor.

THE IMPORTANCE OF "THE SERVE"

Serving drinks is as much about the ritual of building them as anything else. We enjoy something more when we can see it has been made with care and attention to detail; plus, it's nice to take time to prepare something special for the people we host. The right glass and ice, topped off with a great garnish, can transform almost any drink.

The focus of garnish should be on how it smells as well as how it looks. As you tilt that glass to your lips, you'll catch a whiff of the garnish, making for a fuller sensory experience. Think about the flavors in your glass and consider what garnish would bring a complementary aroma.

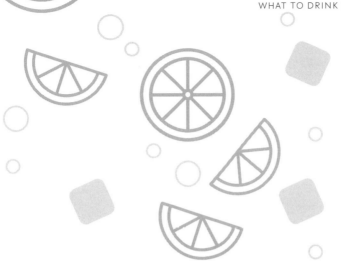

TOP TIPS FOR TONICS AND MIXERS

- **Think about glassware**; it can really add a sense of occasion.
- **Chill everything**. Temperature is key. Tonics and mixers should be chilled and poured over ice. Crushed or cubed, it's up to you.
- **Consider a variety of fruits** such as berries and tropical fruit. Don't just stick to slices of citrus.
- **Use herbs to bring a savory character**. Think beyond rosemary, mint, and thyme to lime leaves and curry leaves.
- **Play at being bartender** and create a fancy rimmed glass. Simply pop some water on a shallow dish, dip the rim of your glass in the water, dip into sugar, and chill. A mix of salt and pepper, instead of the usual sugar, on the rim of a tomato-based drink is superb, too.
- **Be creative.** Enjoy experimenting with new combinations you've never tried before—you'll impress yourself and any guest.

SODAS

When we think of fizzy drinks, the big brands likely spring to mind. While they can be enjoyable, they aren't really the best option for regular consumption. If you've ever witnessed the cleaning power of big-brand cola on a grubby coin, no doubt you'll have considered its effects on your body.

SUGAR AND ADDITIVES

Mainstream brands tend to create oversweetened drinks. They are usually high in sugar and caffeine, which has driven many consumers toward diet and zero versions. But are these artificially sweetened drinks any better for us?

Artificial sweeteners are certainly safe in reasonable amounts for healthy adults—they wouldn't be allowed in food and drink otherwise. But that doesn't make them healthy. For example, there's some evidence that the long-term consumption of diet sodas may not be as effective as you might think in helping with weight loss. That might be psychological rather than physiological—we tell ourselves we've done the right thing having the diet soda, so we feel better about the double cheeseburger with bacon. Simply swapping one drink for another might not be the way forward, particularly if we're not paying attention to the rest of our diet.

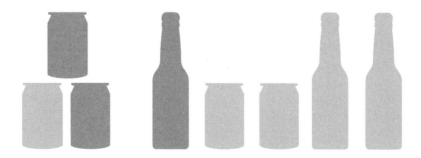

The fact is there are all sorts of flavors, not just sweet ones. Explore a wider range of options and tempt your taste buds away from sugar.

So why recommend sodas at all? Because there are increasing numbers of producers of craft colas, lemonades, and fruit-flavored fizzes who are making drinks with high-quality ingredients and smaller amounts of sugar, letting natural and more subtle flavors shine through.

TOP TIPS FOR SODAS

- **Read the label**. Look for short ingredient lists. If all you find is a jumble of indecipherable numbers and letters, it's probably safe to say that these are things your body could do without.
- **Check the sugar content**. Any fruit-based soda contains naturally occurring sugars, but pay attention to the number of grams of sugar on the drink's label. Four grams is equivalent to 1 teaspoonful of granulated sugar; if you wouldn't eat it, think twice about drinking it.
- **Look for producers who use organic and fair-trade ingredients**, and seek out interesting flavors.
- **Try natural energy drinks** that are rich in guarana or cola nut. These are used around the world as a source of stimulation.
- **Enjoy in moderation**. Consider sodas a treat rather than an everyday drink. It goes without saying that sodas aren't advised for children.

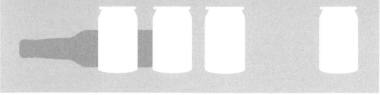

SHRUBS

Shrubs, also known as drinking vinegars, have been around for centuries. They may have first emerged in the Middle East as fruit-based drinks for Muslim populations—certainly the word *sharab* in Arabic means "beverage." But food historians have come across recipes for shrubs in sixteenth-century English texts, as fruit was used to disguise poor-quality alcohol.

Shrubs really rose to prominence in prohibition-era America. Looking for alternatives to the outlawed alcohol, producers began experimenting. Drawing on found recipes, they left fruits to soak in vinegar for several days. Once the fruit was strained out, they mixed the remaining liquid with sugar or honey, and water or soda. This created a drink that balances tartness with sweetness, to be sipped as an alternative to alcohol.

With the end of prohibition, shrubs diminished in popularity. It's only recently that they've enjoyed a resurgence, with commercial-scale production of both syrups and premixed drinks now taking place.

If you are looking for a complex and interesting drink to take the place of alcohol, shrubs come highly recommended from Club Soda members.

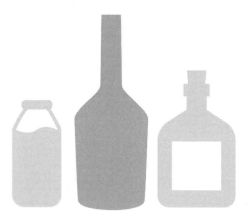

HOW THEY MAKE SHRUBS

The wonderful thing about shrubs is how creative you can be with them. When it comes to ingredients, the only limitation is your imagination. You don't have to stick to just fruits. Herbs and other aromatic plants can be used—foraged rose hips (which are also packed with vitamin C) were used to flavor shrubs in years gone by.

The basic recipe involves mixing the ingredients in a clean jar, where they're muddled to release the juices and aromas, and then covered with raw vinegar. Raw vinegar has not been filtered, and so contains what people call "the mother"—strands of protein, enzymes, and good bacteria. A breathable cloth is placed over the opening of the jar while a short fermentation occurs. Shrubs can be left at room temperature for a few days before straining off the fruit and herbs to leave a liquid that's ready to enjoy.

Because natural yeasts and bacteria are at play, it's important to do your research and handle the process with care.

TOP TIPS FOR SHRUBS

- **Seek out a small, local shrub producer.** A small batch producer is likely to take a great deal of pride and care in making their drinks.
- **Sip slowly.** Savor the quality of ingredients in this grown-up beverage. And try it more than once. Your taste buds will continue to change over time.
- **Embrace the sourness.** Shrubs present a great deal of acidity, though this is balanced by sweet, fruity characters and interesting herbs and spices. If you aren't a fan of sour qualities then shrub may be quite a challenging drink, but it's good to try it at least once.

HOME BREWS

If you're interested in making your own drinks and dabbling in a little kitchen science, then kefir and kombucha may be the perfect match for you. As well as having interesting and complex flavors, these fermented drinks are actually good for you, as they contain beneficial bacteria to support gut health.

Fermented drinks may be all the rage, but some people worry if it's OK to consume them. Like any fermented product, kefir and kombucha contain trace amounts of alcohol, but, because of the presence of bacteria, this can never be in any significant quantity—and certainly not enough to be intoxicating (see also page 142).

What is kefir?

Kefir is a cultured drink, made with milk or water. Water kefir is arguably more useful to the mindful drinker, as it can be more easily mixed with juices, plus it is easier to make in the first place. Kefir has a slight fizz and a gentle sourness. And it's popular because it contains probiotics but no caffeine.

> **"**
> I often used to have a glass of wine beside me when the kids would be doing crafts before dinner. We all have kombucha now.
>
> **Jo**

What is kombucha?

Kombucha is a tea-based drink that's fermented using a SCOBY (a Symbiotic Culture Of Bacteria and Yeast). It is effervescent and has a sour quality. A good-quality kombucha brewed using only tea can still be wonderfully complex.

HOW THEY MAKE KEFIR

Water kefir is made using kefir grains—jellylike beads consisting of bacteria and yeast. Boiling water is added to sugar to dissolve it, and cold water poured in to cool the mixture down. The kefir grains are added. The mixture is then covered and left to ferment at room temperature for 24–48 hours, before being strained for drinking.

Find the grains online; they are reusable indefinitely if cared for.

HOW THEY MAKE KOMBUCHA

The starting ingredient for kombucha is tea (black or green), then sugar, filtered water, and, of course, a SCOBY are needed. Boiling water is added to tea and sugar and left to steep. Once cooled, the SCOBY is added and the whole thing is covered and left to ferment. It is then transferred to an airtight vessel and a little more sugar is added, to taste.

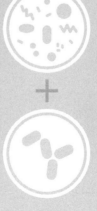

Find kombucha starter kits online, including the all-important SCOBY; there is plenty of further information online for first-time brewers. If you'd rather buy kombucha than make your own, ensure it has been stored in a fridge. If kombucha becomes too hot it can spark more fermentation, resulting in higher acidity, which can be unpleasant.

HOW I CHANGED MY DRINKING: **JUSSI'S STORY**

I started drinking at fourteen, and like most of my friends at school in Finland, we would get as drunk as we could afford to get at least once a week. I even almost learned to like the taste of beer.

As a college student, you were just assumed to drink a lot, so I did. And added the odd weekday night in the pub to all the Fridays and Saturdays at the student union bar.

As I got older, I learned to like not only beer but champagne, whiskey, and cognac, too. The hangovers just got worse and worse though, and the drunken nights less and less fun. I made promises to myself most Sunday mornings to cut down, only to get carried away again come Friday. I decided that I needed to take a complete break, and went teetotal for the first time in my life for a year.

When starting to drink socially again, I did drink less than I used to with only the occasional slip into a major blackout, throwing up in the morning, swearing never-again drunkenness. But those things still happened, no matter how much I swore I would stick to three pints a night and absolutely no more. The third drink was when I forgot my good intentions.

Slowly, over the years, I drank less and less, with a few longer breaks, and felt much better for it. Until one day, having my second small glass of wine, I suddenly thought that I didn't actually enjoy the feeling of getting slightly tipsy. It was quite a shock, as I had always really enjoyed the impact alcohol was having on me. And that, of course, had kept me going for more and more, even though the enjoyable feeling was long gone by the fourth drink.

When I first started on my mindful drinking journey (of course those words didn't even exist back then), the alternatives in most bars were poor to nonexistent. Just sugary soft drinks.

I sometimes wonder how much easier it would have been for me if I'd had the choice that is now available, like all the great low- and no-alcohol beers and other drinks that I've got to know through Club Soda, our Guide, and our Mindful Drinking Festivals.

Where am I now? My daily meditation practice helps me to be mindful, and I'm not quite teetotal, but not far off. I still enjoy the odd glass of wine with a meal or half a pint of ale. But it's been several years since I've last been drunk. And I think I'll keep it like that.

MY STORY:

WHAT I'M DRINKING

THIS SPACE IS FOR YOUR NOTES
ON THE NEW ALCOHOL-FREE DRINKS
YOU'VE TRIED, THE ONES YOU LIKED,
AND THE ONES YOU DIDN'T. MAKE A
NOTE, TOO, OF ANYTHING THAT STANDS
OUT OR IS HELPFUL TO YOU.

These notes pages work alongside pages 140–159. Complete in the spaces below or copy into your journal or notebook.

MY TASTING NOTES

Use the charts below and opposite to keep a track of what you think of each new nonalcoholic drink you try.

THE DRINK	Notes
Taste	
Appearance	
Rating out of 10	

THE DRINK	Notes
Taste	
Appearance	
Rating out of 10	

THE DRINK	Notes
Taste	
Appearance	
Rating out of 10	

THE DRINK	Notes
Taste	
Appearance	
Rating out of 10	

THE DRINK	Notes
Taste	
Appearance	
Rating out of 10	

ADVANCED BEHAVIOR CHANGE

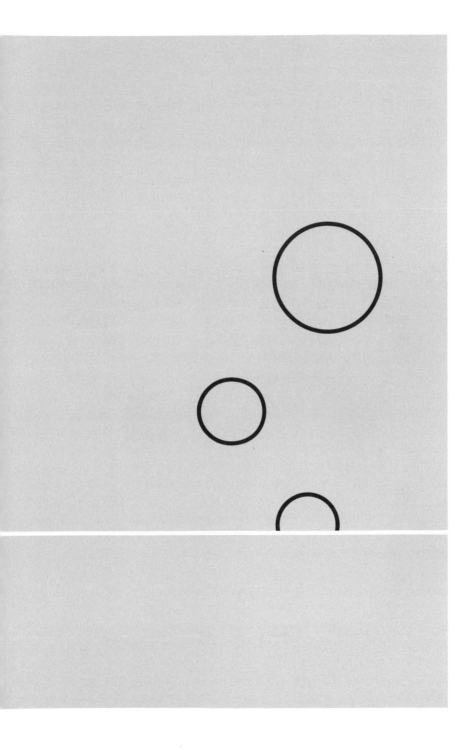

REVIEWING YOUR INTENTIONS

Revisiting your intentions can be one of the most useful things you can do as a mindful drinker (see pages 48 and 66). Change doesn't happen overnight, so you won't want to review your intentions too early in your journey. But every month or so, it can be useful to take a step back, to think about how things are going, and to make some adjustments. Here are some ideas on how to do that.

MULTIDIMENSIONAL INTENTIONS

As you stepped into the different circles of your life and discovered who you want to be (see page 49), you may realize that being a mindful drinker is only incidentally about alcohol. Being a mindful drinker can help you think about the person you want to be, about the roles you want to play in life, about your aspirations for the kind of life you want to have.

In 2019, we carried out some research into Club Soda members' intentions. We found that although our members start with all sorts of different motivations, the most successful mindful drinkers want to change more than their drinking. Their intentions are multidimensional.

So, for example, as well as saying:

> **"I want to have five alcohol-free nights every week."**

They also said things like:

> **"I want to be a better parent."**

> **"I want to feel happier about myself."**

"I want to lose weight."

"I want to be able to focus more at work."

When you change your drinking, having intentions about life changes seems to be more effective than just setting simple goals to limit your alcohol consumption. That's not to say that how much you drink isn't important—whether you're quitting or moderating, it's important to know what you want to achieve. But our research showed that intentions make the biggest difference when they are about your whole life, not just your drinking.

All the different dimensions of your intentions work together to boost your commitment to change.

RETHINK YOUR DRINKING

As you review your intentions, you may realize that the approach you've taken (whether that's cutting down or quitting altogether) isn't quite working. That's OK—you can always rethink the way in which you have changed your drinking (see page 50).

It's too easy to settle for something that doesn't quite work. But changing your approach helps you pay attention again, so you can see afresh the role that alcohol plays in your life. If you've been cutting down but not feeling the benefits, it could be good to go alcohol-free, with or without a time limit.

In the end, being alcohol-free isn't the point, and neither is moderating. Being a mindful drinker is about living the life you imagine and putting alcohol in its proper place, in whatever way works for you.

MOTIVATION

Your reasons for changing your drinking are unique. But if your enthusiasm for change is flagging, it can be useful to understand how motivation generally works. One way that psychologists categorize motivation is by describing it as intrinsic or extrinsic. Here's what they mean by that.

- **If our motivation is intrinsic**, we do something because it is personally rewarding or fulfilling, for its own sake. The motivation comes from within.
- **If our motivation is extrinsic**, we rely on external factors to motivate us, such as rewards (see page 170), punishments, and other people's opinions.

WHAT MOTIVATES YOU?

Many of us have a tendency toward one or other type of motivation to spur us into action. Your decision balance sheet (see page 45) can help you understand what motivates you.

Are your motivations mostly intrinsic, such as wanting to feel differently about yourself or setting yourself a personal challenge? Or are they mostly extrinsic, such as wanting to improve your social status, save money, or perform better at work?

If you're intrinsically motivated, you won't rely on other people's approval; you'll change even if nobody else notices. If you're extrinsically motivated, you'll rely on things outside yourself to get you going. Either way is OK; both types of motivation get the job done.

But understanding your motivation will make a big difference in how you approach rewards (see page 170). If you are strongly intrinsically motivated, external rewards can actually reduce your chances of success. For you, the change is a reward enough in itself. Acknowledge your sense of achievement, but don't damage your motivation by seeking validation from others.

INTRINSIC MOTIVATION BOOSTERS

Because intrinsic motivation is so sensitive to external influence, increasing it is tricky. It's not something you can manipulate directly—after all, you just want to do something or not to some degree—but you can create the space for intrinsic motivation to grow.

Here, the three Cs can help you focus and create new intrinsic motivations to support external ones and to strengthen those you already hold.

THE THREE Cs

Curiosity

You'll want things more if you are curious about them. Whether it's your behavior, your relationships, or your palate, pay closer attention. Dive deeper into change. "I wonder if ..." is an excellent sentence opener to spark curiosity. Try it.

Challenge

Sometimes motivation can dip because things have become too easy. So push yourself. If you haven't yet gone out with your friends alcohol-free, make a date. If there's a new activity that feels a bit scary to try, start it now. Whatever you've been avoiding because it felt too hard, make a plan (see page 52) and start today.

Cooperation

Being a mindful drinker isn't meant to be a solo effort. Sharing your experiences and hearing other people's stories can boost your motivation. And if you're taking on a new challenge, find others who are doing the same—then you can encourage each other.

REWARDS

Rewards are powerful tools for changing your behavior. The promise of a reward—as long as it's the right reward—can be just what you need to begin or to keep going. Rewards are good for motivating you when you don't feel enthusiastic, or if you tend to be extrinsically motivated. But, as we mentioned before, be cautious about rewarding yourself if you're already strongly intrinsically motivated (see page 168).

FINDING NEW REWARDS

Almost anything can be a reward, as long as it meets these four criteria:

- **Purpose** A reward must be special, not something you would do regardless. That's why "going to bed" isn't a reward, but "sleeping in" could be.
- **Proportion** A reward should be in proportion to the effort you've put into attaining it. A spa day might be a great reward to mark one year of mindful drinking, but for one day? Maybe not.
- **Postponement** The reward should come after the task. So keep the alcohol-free fizz on ice until you've achieved what you set out to do.
- **Pleasure** It should go without saying, but your reward should make you happy. Go back to the list of things that make you happy (see pages 92 and 106) and create rewards based on your sensory pleasures.

COUNTING THE DAYS

If you are going alcohol-free in the long term, you might want a reward to tie into particular milestones. One way you could do that is by counting the days.

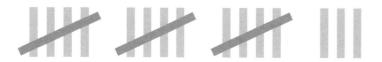

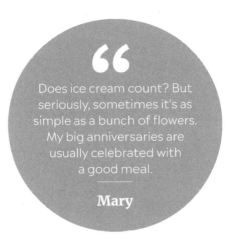

> **"** Does ice cream count? But seriously, sometimes it's as simple as a bunch of flowers. My big anniversaries are usually celebrated with a good meal.
>
> **Mary**

Counting acts like a reward because you turn passing time into a number. As that number grows, it becomes an ever-increasing reward. Seeing the days add up can reinforce your sense of achievement.

Bear in mind, though, that while you're creating such a reward, you can also experience the reverse—an escalating punishment hanging over you. The loss of that number—especially if it's a big number—might feel devastating. That fear could keep you going, if other motivations fail. But what happens if things don't go according to plan? Whether it's a minor slip-up or a train wreck, do you have to restart at day one?

The simple answer is no. Whether you stuck to your intentions for 3 days or 30 years, that time still matters. If yesterday went according to plan and today didn't, it doesn't mean that yesterday wasn't worthwhile. Congratulate yourself on the days you lived well and get back on track (see page 194).

The time may come when counting doesn't help any more as a motivational reward. And one day you'll wake up and realize you've lost count, and that day, in particular, is a day to reward yourself.

HABITS

Habits are things that we do repeatedly and, most of the time, unconsciously. We often think of habits as bad things to be broken. But once we understand how and why the brain forms habits, we can start to use them for good.

THE ANATOMY OF A HABIT

Ultimately, the brain is lazy: if it can create a shortcut to save expending energy, it will. This is why your brain forms habits.

Habits have three parts:

TRIGGER
For instance, walking into your kitchen when
you come home from work

ROUTINE
The pouring of a glass of wine

PAYOFF
In this case, the feeling of relaxation you
associate with drinking alcohol.

The payoff is especially important because it incentivizes your brain to make the routine automatic, and it leaves you with a craving so you're ready to respond to the next trigger that comes along (see pages 186–189).

USING HABITS FOR GOOD

You don't need to banish bad habits. Instead, use your understanding of their anatomy to repurpose them. Pay attention to your triggers (see page 186) and use them to build new routines to give you good feelings (see page 92).

A good place to start is disrupting the routine. Going back to the example opposite, you could move the wine rack to another room. Or you could put a big note on your fridge door with a reminder to drink a glass of water. Or you could completely remove alcohol from your home.

It's important to remember that the payoff isn't the bottle of wine itself, but the feeling that comes with it. The real payoff at the end of the habit routine isn't a physical reward. A feeling of relaxation might seem less tangible and harder to grasp, but it really matters. So skip the wine and go straight for the feeling itself. You could, for example, write the word "calm" on your kitchen door and leave a scented candle on the counter, ready to light when you get home.

How else could you jolt a lazy brain out of its comfortable patterns?

Once you've begun paying attention to your habits, you can begin playing with them. Be creative. Experiment with new approaches to routines—for example, by building chains of tiny habits that follow one another, as automatically as you wash your hands after going to the bathroom.

And identify what are known as your "keystone" habits—these habits have an impact on multiple areas of your life, and they create the conditions for other positive habits to flourish. While they might not appear particularly significant at first glance, you notice the difference if they don't happen. Often, they are important to setting up a good day, such as meditation, a nourishing breakfast, or a quiet cup of coffee.

Once you're happy with new habits, it takes time and repetition for them to become truly automatic. Some people say 21 days, but it really takes as long as it takes for them to become unconscious patterns of behavior. At some point, your lazy brain will take these new habits on board and they will support you to live the life you imagine.

DISTRACTIONS

We have a confession to make. We haven't told you the whole truth.

We didn't want to tell you this before now because it could have been confusing. But now you've come to grips with mindful drinking, we think you'll understand. We buried this secret here, deep within the book, so only those people who get this far will discover it.

Are you ready? Take a deep breath. Here we go.

Mindfulness doesn't always work.

Actually, it's more than that. There are times in life when mindfulness can actually make things worse.

NOT PAYING ATTENTION

One of the strange gifts alcohol gave us was the power to ignore anything. Whether it was our troublesome emotions, intrusive thoughts, or social anxiety, we could simply switch off.

As a mindful drinker, there are also going to be times when, legitimately, you will want to *not* pay attention. When you crave a drink but don't know what to do about it (see page 188). When you feel a sense of discomfort but you're too tired to figure out why. When you want so badly to hit the "f*ck it" button (see page 192), and you aren't sure if you can hold yourself back.

In those moments, mindfulness is going to make things worse, because whatever is going on will feel more intense and overwhelming when you approach it mindfully. Fortunately, your brain has a limited capacity for focus, so if you can keep it busy for a while, you will start to feel better.

All will be well. But to get there, you'll have to temporarily forget everything you've learned about mindfully paying attention.

THE IDEAL DISTRACTION

To work well as a distraction, an activity:

- requires just enough concentration to give your brain something to do, but it shouldn't feel like hard work
- is simple—make sure it's not emotionally demanding—such as a game on your phone, a knitting pattern, a coloring book, a crossword puzzle, or a sitcom box set (download episodes to your phone for instant access)

You may already know your ideal distraction. Do you ever find yourself lost in an activity, not knowing where the time went but feeling strangely content? Think of it as being "in the flow"—where everything else apart from what you're doing simply falls away into the background. If you experience such feelings then that activity is your ideal distraction.

Whatever you think your distraction activity is, test it in advance to make sure it works. Then keep your resources, whatever they may be, somewhere within easy reach for any emergency.

Using your distraction isn't a tactic for every day, but it's best to be prepared for those days when applying mindfulness techniques is not going to help. When the reason to distract yourself has passed, you'll be thankful for being a little bit "mindless" for a while.

> " I enjoy a challenge, so I set myself the task of finding an activity that doesn't require boozing for each letter of the alphabet.
>
> **Jen**

BRYNN EXPERIMENTED WITH CHANGING
AND FOUND WHAT WORKS FOR HER

HOW I CHANGED MY DRINKING: **BRYNN'S STORY**

Work drinking is an integral part of my workplace, which you might not expect seeing as I am a schoolteacher. But you're with kids all week long and the first thing everyone wants to do come Friday night is go hit the bar.

For the longest time I had a routine: Monday through Thursday, work very hard, sleep a little bit, end the week exhausted. Friday night, we would all go to the same bar, get very drunk, very early. Wake up feeling like trash on Saturday. Do it all again Saturday night. Feel like trash on Sunday. And then go and do it all again.

One Friday, there was a new teacher at the bar, and I noticed he didn't drink the whole time. He told me he was six months sober. And the more he told me about his journey, the more I realized that I was having a lot of the same problems that he had. Our friendship really took off from there, and that's where this all started.

For me, changing has been a very slow process. Very trial and error, very up and down. Midway through 2017, I told myself that I was going to go for four months without drinking and give it a test run. After that, I decided to dip my foot back in the drinking pool for a while. But I went through these cycles where things would go badly. I would have a plan to go out and have two drinks, but for whatever reason, things would go off the rails.

Whenever I would mess up, some people would give me reassurances that it was completely normal. But Club Soda is full of people who are mirroring this new habit of mine. I'd take some time, and realize that I didn't have to feel this way right now. It had all been in my control if I chose to see it that way. I had to look in the mirror and be honest with myself.

Now, I understand those plans to have a couple of drinks don't work for me. I know they work for many people, but they just don't work for me, at least at this point in my life.

At the end of 2018, I decided that I would give myself at least one full calendar year off booze, and I was about six months in when I just decided that's probably going to be the way that it stays.

My life at this moment is by no means perfect but, in many ways, I wake up every day feeling almost like I'm living in a dream. I'm living in my heaven now.

MY STORY:
CHANGING MY
BEHAVIOR

THIS SPACE IS FOR NOTES ON YOUR
MOTIVATIONS, WHAT REWARDS WORK,
BUILDING NEW HABITS, AND IDENTIFYING
YOUR IDEAL DISTRACTIONS.

These notes pages work alongside the prompts across pages 168–175
Complete in the spaces below or copy into your journal or notebook.

MOTIVATION

Explore your intrinsic motivations (see also page 168–169). Write down what
you think these are:

I will build my intrinsic motivation by asking myself ...

What am I curious about?

What's challenging me?

Who can I cooperate with, and about what?

REWARDS

Remembering that a reward must meet all of the following criteria—purpose, proportion, postponement, and pleasure (see also pages 170–171)—what could be your ideal reward?

HABITS

Explore your habits and break them down into triggers, routines, and payoffs, so you can start to build new ones (see also pages 172–173).

What habits do I notice? (Good or bad, I won't judge myself.)

Once you've identified the habits (above), try to work out how they break down under the headings below.

TRIGGER	ROUTINE	PAYOFF

DISTRACTIONS

Having a "bank" of mindless distractions can help you cope with situations that are potentially overwhelming (see also pages 174–175).

What are my ideal distraction activities?

> **"**
>
> For my one year anniversary, I got gifts from my mom and dad—but seeing them proud of their daughter again was the biggest reward.
>
> **Claire**

PRACTICAL PROBLEM SOLVING

WITHDRAWAL // TRIGGERS // CRAVINGS //
AMBIVALENCE // THE "F*CK IT" BUTTON //
GETTING BACK ON TRACK // SARAH'S STORY //
MY STORY: SOLVING MY PROBLEMS

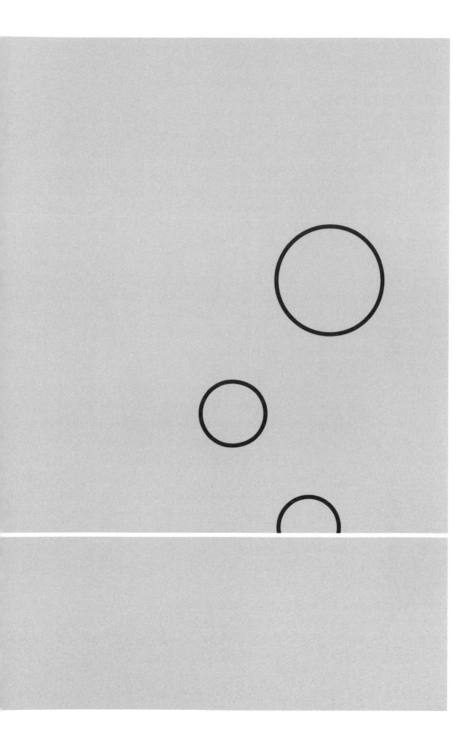

WITHDRAWAL

If you've turned to this page directly from the introduction (see page 13), you may be worried that you are physically dependent on alcohol.

WHAT PHYSICAL DEPENDENCE MEANS

Unlike other drugs, alcohol actually becomes part of how our bodies work. Our tolerance for alcohol rises over time. When we first started drinking, we felt drunk after one or two drinks. Now, it might take four or more. If we rarely feel drunk, that's because our bodies have become accustomed to alcohol. Tolerance isn't the same as physical dependence, but it's a sign that our bodies are learning to cope with alcohol's persistent presence. This isn't a good thing, as it increases our risk of becoming physically dependent on alcohol.

Physical dependence means that the body has become so used to alcohol that it actually needs it to work normally. If we drink every day for a long time, and especially if we need a drink to feel emotionally or physically OK, we might have become physically dependent on alcohol. And if we are physically dependent and then suddenly stop drinking, the body cannot react quickly enough to be able to deal with the absence of alcohol. That's when withdrawal symptoms kick in.

WITHDRAWAL SYMPTOMS

The mildest withdrawal symptoms include sweating, shakes, headaches, and nausea. Some people might feel anxious or agitated. At their most severe, symptoms include seizures and delirium tremens (otherwise known as the DTs)—a rapid onset of delusions, hallucinations, and vomiting.

Hangovers get better within hours; withdrawal symptoms get worse and can last for days or weeks. If your symptoms don't improve, seek medical help. In rare cases, alcohol withdrawal can be fatal.

You also might experience what's known as post-acute withdrawal symptoms, such as mood swings, sleep disturbances, and memory problems. These symptoms can come in waves over several years, and they are a sign that your body is healing itself. Don't worry—they will pass by themselves— but do seek help if you need it (see page 208).

WORRYING ABOUT WITHDRAWAL

It's important to put all of this in perspective. Fewer than 2 percent of adults are physically dependent on alcohol.

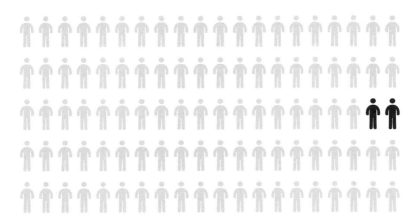

Of those, only 5-10 percent of physically dependent drinkers ever experience a seizure or delirium tremens. So don't let worry about withdrawal hold you back from changing your drinking.

Talk to your doctor (see page 208). Unless you have been drinking heavily, they are unlikely to recommend the hospital or rehab. Most alcohol withdrawal happens safely at home, through a gradual reduction in consumption.

Getting to the other side of alcohol withdrawal is just the first step. There's an exciting journey ahead of you to become a mindful drinker.

TRIGGERS

If you've been thinking about your habits (see page 172), you might have already identified some of your triggers for drinking.

But triggers don't just spark the automatic behavior we spoke of before. Sometimes, a trigger can itself lead to a craving for a drink (see page 188). If you're going to stick to your mindful drinking plans, you'll need to find ways to identify potential triggers and know how to deal with them.

WHAT TRIGGERS YOU?

We recently asked Club Soda members about triggers, and the diversity of responses was incredible. They ranged from the obvious—Friday night with the kids tucked up in bed—to the obscure—an episode of *The Archers*. Some were triggered at certain times of the day, while for others it was particular places and people. Takeout, vacations, smoking, or airports ... almost anything, it seems, could be a trigger.

What are your triggers? Keep track of them (see page 198). The questions you learned to pay attention to your drinking (see pages 24–27) can help you:

- **Where?** Are there certain places or particular situations in which you feel the urge to drink?
- **When?** Are there particular times of day, days of the week, vacations, or events that trigger you?
- **Who?** Are there people around whom you're more likely to feel triggered?
- **What?** Are there particular things that trigger you? What else can you think of that acts as a trigger?

Having identified your triggers, next you can set about making a plan for how best to deal with them.

DEALING WITH TRIGGERS

There are three basic ways to handle any trigger: avoidance, control, or escape.

Avoidance

If a trigger is ongoing, it may be easiest to avoid it altogether. If you associate your favorite TV show with having a drink, for example, are you willing to stop watching it? How could you replace the good feelings you associated with it? Bear in mind that getting rid of a trigger can result in feelings of loss.

Control

There are some triggers you might not want to remove from your life. Control isn't about trying to change the trigger, but rather altering your response to it. The skills you learned for if–then planning can help (see page 57). If, for instance, you identify that being angry is a trigger for wanting to drink, you can learn to recognize that emotion and find new ways of expressing your feelings that don't involve reaching for a bottle.

Escape

Sometimes a trigger catches you off guard. If you can't avoid a known trigger and you don't control your response, escape is the best plan. Leave the situation; put some actual distance between you and the trigger.

Escape is like an unplanned moment of avoidance. Learn from the experience; next time, you'll deal with the trigger better.

> "
> It's not one thing—environment and people and mood all contribute. I found I could rank these and make plans for the most difficult combinations.
>
> **Emma**

CRAVINGS

We've discovered that a trigger sets up the potential for a drink (see page 186). A craving, though, is the feeling that we really want that drink. Right now!

Cravings can arise without a trigger and they can take you by surprise. Weeks could have gone by since you last thought about having a drink and then, seemingly out of nowhere, you find yourself craving. Cravings are not unusual. If you feel a craving, there's nothing wrong with you.

WHAT EXACTLY IS A CRAVING?

A craving is a sudden and strong desire for something. That definition can help you put your cravings into perspective. A faint urge isn't a craving. If it's been and gone in moments, it wasn't a craving. Don't let it bother you.

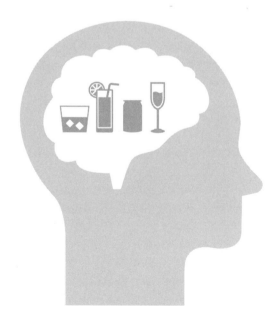

But some desires are persistent and can feel overwhelming. You might even experience a craving physically—a knot in the stomach or dry mouth. However unpleasant it is in the short term, know that the craving will pass.

SURFING THE URGE

When you feel a craving, it can be tempting to struggle with it. But tackling it head-on and trying to make it go away can, in fact, make it worse.

There is a specific mindfulness technique for dealing with cravings known as "urge surfing." The name is evocative, for good reason: imagine the craving as a wave that bobs you up and down as it heads to shore. It will pass and the sea will be calm again. However big the wave, you just have to wait it out.

Try this when you feel a craving:
- Close your eyes and focus on breathing calmly and slowly—in and out, in and out.
- Remind yourself that, even as the craving increases, it will ebb away.
- Notice the craving and let it go; it will pass.
- Continue to focus on your breathing until your sense of calm returns.

EATING MATTERS

Cravings aren't just in your head—they can have a physical component, too. One of the reasons you might be prone to cravings is hunger (see page 102).

If you are feeling cravings often, keep a food diary. Notice what and when you eat, and when you feel cravings for a drink. Changing the patterns of your eating and the quality of your food could help control your cravings.

AMBIVALENCE

It's normal to feel ambivalent about change.

We want to change, but there's a part of us that wants to cling to the past. This state is part of the process of change. If every part of us were ready to go, we would have changed already.

Ambivalence feels like the moment just before we take the next step.

But it isn't always obvious. Sometimes, ambivalence can be lurking inside the issues that we choose to ignore. Avoiding a difficult decision can be a sign that the factors we need to consider are finely balanced. Equally, ambivalence can manifest itself as procrastination, that state of never quite getting around to doing something you've been meaning to do. This could be a sign of needing to dive deeper into the pros and cons of the issue.

REVISIT YOUR "WHY?"

Remember the decision balance sheet (see pages 35 and 44)? This tool to discover your motivations is useful again now. Things may well have changed since you became a mindful drinker, so it's useful to revisit your initial motivations—and redo a decision balance sheet—to see what's different.

Often, what underlies ambivalence is a worry that the cost of making a positive change is too high. The decision balance sheet can help you think this through; turn to page 200 and complete a new version. As before, remember to be honest, be brave, and be as specific as possible.

- Start by identifying what it is that you feel ambivalent about.
- Map out the pros and cons of changing, as well as the pros and cons of staying the same.
- Don't give each of the items a score this time—that would only confirm to you how finely balanced the argument is.
- Look specifically at the reasons to change and the reasons why you don't want to stay the same. What can you do to strengthen these factors? Are there any benefits you've overlooked? How can you shift the balance toward positive action?

FLIP A COIN

If ambivalence gets out of hand, don't get stuck going round in circles. Instead, flip a coin (or use some other divination method). Deliberately taking away your power to choose and presenting one of the two options to yourself as a done deal will quickly tell you if you can really live with the consequences.

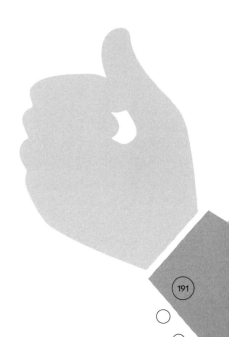

Decide which option is heads and which is tails. Clear your mind. Take a breath. Then flip.

Got heads, but really wanted tails? Then go for tails. Still stuck?

If all else fails, just do something. It's better than doing nothing.

THE "F*CK IT" BUTTON

You can stop your mindful drinking journey dead in its tracks. In Club Soda, we call this hitting the "f*ck it" button.

We use this admittedly colorful language because of how hitting the button feels. We hit the "f*ck it" button, knowing it could undermine our progress, and that we might put ourselves in an even worse position. But we simply don't care. It's the ultimate act of self-sabotage.

SELF-SABOTAGE

When we sabotage ourselves, we're not just messing up our intentions and plans. Self-sabotage damages us. So why on earth would we want to do this? Psychologists suggest a wide range of reasons, including:

- lack of self-worth
- worrying that we are frauds
- a tendency to blame ourselves
- the familiarity of failure
- sheer boredom.

Any of these things might be true, but we'd like to suggest another reason we hit the "f*ck it" button. Deep down, we'd rather have the shitty certainty of our old lives than face the wild unknown of the future.

REMEMBERING THE PAST

If there's one thing to be said in favor of life before we started becoming a mindful drinker, at least it was predictable. Spending Saturdays on the sofa nursing a hangover wasn't so bad, was it? Those long drinking sessions with friends were fun, weren't they?

Rosy retrospection is a common human experience, and it's not that we actively choose to misremember. The lazy brain, as we've met before

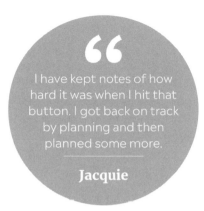

"
I have kept notes of how
hard it was when I hit that
button. I got back on track
by planning and then
planned some more.

Jacquie

(see page 172), compresses and simplifies memories, discarding whatever it can. It turns out a human brain isn't quite up to the task of remembering the entirety of a human life. So, instead of trusting your memories, trust this fact: **at some point, a past version of you was convinced that you had to change**. And so you began.

TRUSTING TODAY

Trust isn't blind optimism. It's actually born out of the reality of your experiences. Whatever else has happened, you have survived up to this point in your life. However difficult things have been, somehow you've kept going. You might even have thrived and been happy. Of course, the past isn't a predictor of the future, but today doesn't feel so different to yesterday, does it? Tomorrow is likely to be much the same.

So it's important to hold your nerve, and trust. What you trust in is less important than the act of trusting. Even a suggestion that everything will work out manages to defuse the "f*ck it" button.

GETTING BACK ON TRACK

Something got the better of you, despite your mindful drinking intentions; your plans fell by the wayside. You drank a lot more than you wanted to.

Don't worry, it's all going to be OK.

DEALING WITH HANGOVERS

First things first, let's deal with the hangover you might be experiencing. If it's been a while since your last one, you might be feeling particularly rough. There have been thousands of studies on the physiological effects of getting drunk, but only a handful on what actually causes hangovers. None of them has found a foolproof cure, so this is our best advice:

• Prioritize your physical needs: sleep if you need to; sip water if you are dehydrated but feel queasy; take painkillers for a headache; and eat some nutritious food when you can manage it.

• Don't drink any more booze; the "hair of the dog" remedy is not advisable.

• Don't drive. If you drank a lot and woke up without a hangover, you may still be drunk.

WHAT HAPPENED?

As the hangover starts to pass, you might reflect and feel like you've let yourself down, but actually you've given yourself an amazing learning opportunity.

Ask yourself the questions that help you pay attention to your drinking (see pages 24–27). But remember not to ask "why?"—that can quickly lead to beating yourself up. If shame creeps up on you, banish it with an outpouring of self-care. Treat yourself kindly, as you would a friend.

Try to piece together what happened. Identify the moment things started going wrong. Maybe you fell into an old habit (see page 172) or missed a trigger (see page 186)? Or did you hit the "f*ck it" button (see page 192)?

To get to the bottom of the story, it can be helpful to ask yourself:

- Where was I? If I went out, did I go to a number of different places? Or was I at home? Or somewhere else?
- When did it happen? When did I start drinking? What happened next? Are there moments that stand out? Or moments I can't remember?
- Who was I with? In a big group? On my own?

Remember, this isn't about blaming anyone, including you. You're just paying attention to what happened.

It's possible that you have big gaps in your memory. Blackouts are a type of amnesia caused by drinking so quickly that your brain loses its ability to form memories. Knowing this is useful information in itself. But don't dwell on the gaps, focus on what you can recall.

As you zero in on the moment it started going wrong, remember that you are learning. Ask yourself what you could have done differently. How could you avoid the situation next time around? Incorporate these discoveries into new if-then plans (see page 57).

Most of all, don't worry. These things happen to the best of us. Pick up your intentions right where you left them. The life you want is still waiting for you.

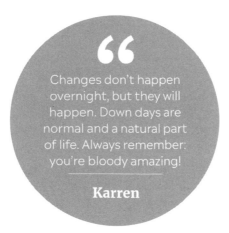

> " Changes don't happen overnight, but they will happen. Down days are normal and a natural part of life. Always remember: you're bloody amazing!
>
> **Karren**

SARAH IS A BARTENDER WHO FOUND
HER OWN WAY TO CHANGE

HOW I CHANGED MY DRINKING: **SARAH'S STORY**

It started when I got my first and only DUI. I didn't injure anybody or hurt myself, but I got pulled over because I was going too slow. In many states, if you get a DUI you can opt to take "alcohol classes." You have to stay sober throughout the entire time, and they're very expensive—but it's either that or jail time.

So I had to attend AA and I was sober for seven months. I hadn't identified as an alcoholic and I didn't believe that I was an alcoholic. I thought I was just having a really rough patch. But soon I felt better, physically and mentally. Then I started drinking again, because I thought, "I got this, I can do this normally." But I can't. There is no casual drinking for me anymore.

Later, when I stopped drinking of my own accord, I went back to AA for a while. But I realized that while I'd learned a lot from it, there are different routes to recovery. Instagram helped me. I found accounts like Club Soda to follow. At first, it was nice to find people saying "I've been there, I know how that feels." That's when I started using it as a tool, a community of people I could lean on and say

"Hey, I'm having this kind of day, what do I do?"

My fiancé still drinks. In the beginning, there were a couple of times when I was like "Hey, your beer smells really good, you gotta get away!" But I feel very fortunate that I've been able to draw a line. I have told him, though, that whiskey is not allowed in our house, and we don't have beer in the refrigerator. If he decides that he wants to have a couple of beers after work, he will stop at the store, then come home and have them and that will be it.

It's different for everybody, but I don't drink alcohol-free beers either. I worry that it could trigger me into drinking actual beer. I haven't had anything in my mouth that tastes like alcohol for two and a half years, and that's a distinction that I have to make.

I took a break from bartending when I first stopped drinking, but I came back to it. I think that I'm better at my job now because I am so much more with it and I see the things that people do. It keeps it real for me and it helps me remember. And I get nice little reminders of those behaviors that I don't want to have in my life ever again.

MY STORY:
SOLVING MY PROBLEMS

THIS SPACE IS FOR NOTES ON YOUR TRIGGERS, AMBIVALENCE, AND GETTING BACK ON TRACK. JOT DOWN ANYTHING ELSE THAT IS IMPORTANT TO YOU, TOO.

These notes pages work alongside the prompts across pages 186–195. Complete in the spaces below or copy into your journal or notebook.

TRIGGERS

It can help to apply these questions to identify your triggers (see also pages 186–187). Make a note, too, if you can avoid, control, or escape them.

WHERE?	Avoid	Control	Escape

WHEN?	Avoid	Control	Escape

WHO?	Avoid	Control	Escape

WHAT?	Avoid	Control	Escape

AMBIVALENCE

If you're feeling ambivalent about the mindful drinking changes you've made, revisit your motivations using the blank decision balance sheet below (see also pages 190–191). But remember not to add any scores this time.

MY DECISION BALANCE SHEET	UPSIDES (what will be good, benefits, gains)	DOWNSIDES (what will be difficult, risks, losses)
Staying the same (not changing drinking)		
Changing drinking		

How can I strengthen my motivations to change?

GETTING BACK ON TRACK

Ask yourself some questions to piece together what happened when you drank more than you wanted to. It's a great experience to learn from.

Where was I?

When did it happen?

Who was I with?

MY NEW IF-THEN PLANS

This is what I'll do next time:

IF	THEN

WHAT'S NEXT?

BEING A MINDFUL DRINKER // FINDING
THE OTHERS // ASKING FOR HELP // KEEPING
GOING // LOOKING BACK, LOOKING FORWARD //
DRU'S STORY // MY STORY: WHAT'S NEXT FOR ME?

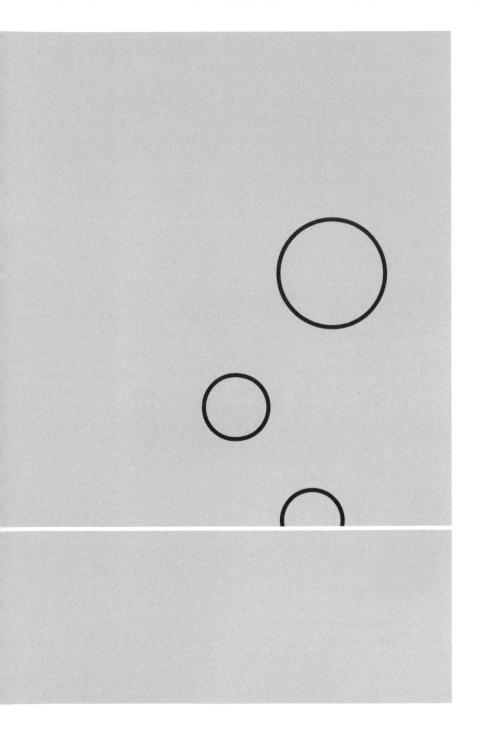

BEING A MINDFUL DRINKER

If you've worked through this book and changed your drinking as a result, you have done an extraordinary thing. Of course, things haven't always gone according to plan. But don't let what went wrong overshadow the enormous number of things that have gone right. You deserve to feel proud of yourself.

As you approach the end of this book, this last chapter is about what's next. Now you've done the hard work of changing, how do you keep hold of all the benefits of becoming who you are?

SHIFTING YOUR IDENTITY

Behavior-change experts working with people who quit smoking say there's a moment when an ex-smoker becomes a nonsmoker.

That might look at first glance like a semantic difference, but it points to something much deeper. A behavior that has defined someone, sometimes for much of their life, suddenly stops being the most important thing about them. Their new "nonsmoker" identity makes their commitment to changing unshakably real. It fundamentally redefines them as a person, and signals that something truly profound has happened. They've become who they are.

Whatever part you've decided alcohol is going to play in your life, there's a shift in identity that's waiting for you, a new story that's waiting to be told.

You're not just someone who has stopped or changed their drinking. You are a mindful drinker.

Taking on a new identity can feel awkward at first. And sometimes, it can take a while before it feels like us. So try this. Stand in front of your mirror, look yourself squarely in the eye, and say:

"I am a mindful drinker."

COMING OUT

It's possible that you have undertaken this journey quietly and entirely alone. If you have, now might be the time to change that. As you become confident in your identity as a mindful drinker, you'll want to share it with the world, too. Imagine:

- telling your friends and family you are a mindful drinker
- turning down an unwanted drink saying: "No thanks, I'm a mindful drinker"
- walking into a bar and asking what they have for mindful drinkers.

OK, we'll admit it. "Mindful drinker" isn't a common phrase yet, so it might take some explanation at first. But mindful drinking is something that more and more people are talking about. And when it comes to changing your drinking, you've always been a trailblazer.

Wherever you go, be an active customer. If you want pubs and bars to stay open where you live, stay friends with them. They appreciate your continued patronage, whatever you are drinking. They want to know what will keep you coming back, so ask them to stock your favorite nonalcoholic drinks (see pages 146–159). The Club Soda Guide at clubsodaguide.com lists hundreds of alcohol-free drinks, so you know what you can find where. So, if you're looking for an amazing alcohol-free night out, the Guide is a great place to start. If you discover a great venue, you can nominate it for inclusion in the Guide at clubsodaguide.com.

Being a mindful drinker isn't just about changing your drinking. It's about changing the world around you, so you make it easier for other people to become mindful drinkers, too.

That's why we say that Club Soda is a mindful drinking movement.

FINDING THE OTHERS

One day, we'll live in a world where anyone can walk into any bar and order whatever they like, and drink it in the company of people who don't bat an eyelid about their choices. Until that time, there's safety in numbers.

As you've become a mindful drinker, you might have realized that you don't want to socialize with old drinking buddies all the time. Your old social life was a perfect fit for the person you were, but you might need some new people around you as you become who you are. The good news is that there are other mindful drinkers out there, just like you. All you have to do is find them.

Making new friends who enjoy the things you do can take time. But there's a world of alcohol-free activities for you to explore, and places where you can make friends. From foreign language meetups to walking groups, many mindful drinkers have built amazing social lives without alcohol. Whether you become a volunteer, take a pottery class, or join a cycling club, it's great to get to know people in environments that don't make getting drunk a necessity.

JOIN CLUB SODA

Whatever stage you've reached in changing your drinking and becoming who you are, there's a place for you in Club Soda.

There are Club Soda members hanging on the edge of the conversation, wondering if they are ready to take the plunge, right through to people who have happily been mindful drinkers for years. There are even members who have never drunk alcohol at all and just like hanging out with us. Some of us

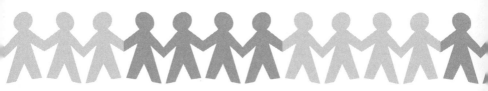

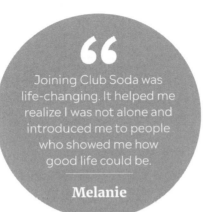

> "
> Joining Club Soda was
> life-changing. It helped me
> realize I was not alone and
> introduced me to people
> who showed me how
> good life could be.
>
> **Melanie**

are alcohol-free, others of us are moderating, and a few of us don't really go for hard definitions of our drinking style. We don't like labels.

Whoever you are, being a Club Soda member means you're part of a gang that gets you. We're great at offering support and encouragement. We know that there's life beyond drinking. If you want to dive deeper, Club Soda has a blog full of advice on more subjects than we could cram into this book. We run online courses and real-world workshops to build skills and confidence to help you change. Whether you want to take a month off booze or join a longer-term program, we've got the support you need to become who you are.

And there's more. We've got a guide to pubs, bars, and restaurants. And we run festivals, events, and lunches if you want to meet others face-to-face.

Come and find us at joinclubsoda.com.

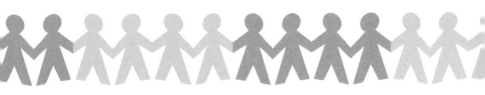

ASKING FOR HELP

It's OK to need help. Sometimes, socializing with others (see page 112) and the support we can get from friends (see page 116) just aren't enough to help us deal with the issues we are facing. We are trying our best, but we realize we can't do it alone.

We feel like we are trying to walk through quicksand. We need someone who knows how to get unstuck.

Reaching this point can feel like an admission of failure, as if you weren't up to the task of changing by yourself. Be reassured that you are not the first person to need help from a professional, and you won't be the last. You're in good company. Asking for help can be a supreme act of courage, and it might just be the best thing you've ever done for yourself.

FINDING SUPPORT

Club Soda doesn't run face-to-face support groups, but if you want to join one, we recommend Smart Recovery. It's not just for alcohol, but for drugs, gambling and other addictive behaviors, too. Grounded in science, Smart Recovery can help you build motivation, cope with urges, manage your thoughts, and live a balanced life.

smartrecovery.org

SPECIALIST SERVICES

- **Alcohol treatment**: Lots of rehab and detox centers advertise, but they vary in quality and cost. The best gateway to specialized local alcohol support and treatment is your doctor. They can help you find the services in your area that are best for you.

- **Counseling and therapy**: There are several nationwide directories of counselors and therapists, so you can find the support you need, from anxiety to relationship issues. Ensure any counselor or therapist is licenced, and supportive of your approach to changing your drinking. Ask if they accept your insurance, too. The 2008 mental health parity law requires coverage of services for mental health and substance-use disorders to be comparable to physical health coverage, so check your insurance plan.

psychologytoday.com/us/therapists

goodtherapy.org

- **Financial issues**: If you are struggling with debt or other financial problems, the National Foundation for Credit Counseling can help.

  Visit nfcc.org or call 1-800-388-2227

- **Legal issues**: Free or low-cost legal help can be hard to find, but usa.gov/legal-aid is a good place to start looking if you need advice.

- **Mental health**: In a crisis, call the National Suicide Prevention Lifeline at 1-800-273-8255 or you can chat online at suicidepreventionlifeline.org/chat. The Lifeline provides 24/7 free and confidential support.

- **Sexual assault**: RAINN (Rape, Abuse & Incest National Network) is the biggest anti-sexual violence organization in the US, and operates the National Sexual Assault Hotline. Call 1-800-656-4673 or go to rainn.org.

Help with alcohol withdrawal

Caution: for physically dependent drinkers, alcohol withdrawal without medical support can be dangerous.

If you think you might be physically dependent on alcohol, you must talk to your doctor. Your doctor can assess your risk and give you advice about how to stop safely. Until then, it's safer to keep drinking while you wait for a doctor's appointment. You can still read this book and think about how you want to change, but do not stop drinking suddenly.

KEEPING GOING

A time will come when the act of changing your drinking will be a distant memory. Being a mindful drinker will be such an ordinary part of who you are, you'll barely give it any thought.

Some people worry that it's dangerous to reach this point. If we drop our guard, even for a moment, we might find ourselves back where we started. It only takes one drink. That, at least, is the story you've told yourself. Like any story, you don't have to believe it (see page 31).

To be clear, nobody can predict your future. There are no studies of people who have changed their drinking that can tell you your chances of sticking with it for the long term. But why believe the worst will happen, when you could believe the best? You've come this far, and you can keep going. And you can be confident that the longer you do something, the more likely you are to continue.

NEVER STOP BELIEVING

Of course, things do go tragically wrong for some people. Everyone's heard a story of someone who spent years, maybe even decades, on the straight and narrow, who falls back into heavy drinking with terrible and self-destructive consequences. If that person was a celebrity, we might read newspaper headlines about them. The media loves a tragic hero, after all. You might have come across those stories and thought to yourself: "You see, I told you so. People can't really change." But it's important to know that these cases are vanishingly rare, which is why we hear about them. People happily living their lives don't make newspaper headlines. And there are more people happily living their lives than you can possibly imagine.

If, years later, you have a slip-up, don't turn it into a disaster. One bad day doesn't undo years of progress. It's just a bad day, and you can bounce back from it. Take care of yourself, and get back on track (see page 194). If you've been counting days, you don't have to restart at day one (see page 171). But priorities will have changed, so revisit your intentions and think about who you want to become now (see page 166). Just because you've changed your drinking, you don't have to stop changing. Now might be your best time to grow.

LOOK HOW FAR YOU'VE COME!

Every now and again, stop and look back. There's a path made of your steps that leads right to your feet. As you look at the trail you've made, you'll notice the ups and downs, the places you got stuck, and the giant leaps forward. But you might not be able to see all the way to where you began any more.

Step by step, you've found yourself in a completely new place. And you realize you couldn't go back to the life you lived before, even if you tried.

It's OK to feel sad about this, as well as happy. It's a normal part of changing to leave old versions of yourself behind; think of it like a skin you shed. Remember who you were with deep gratitude. You wouldn't be who you are today if you hadn't lived your life.

It's good where you've been, and it's also good where you're going.

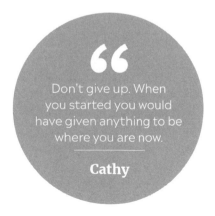

Don't give up. When you started you would have given anything to be where you are now.

Cathy

LOOKING BACK, LOOKING FORWARD

Here we are. At the end. Can you believe it? Think of everything that's happened since you picked up this book and began working your way through it. Think of everything that's changed, not least you.

You've done an amazing thing for yourself in becoming a mindful drinker. But this part of your journey is coming to an end.

REFLECTION AND PLANNING

It's good to look back and remember, and it's good to look forward and dream. Below are some questions to help you reflect on your experiences and plan for what comes next (see pages 216–219). So find a quiet corner. Pour yourself your favorite alcohol-free drink. Open your journal. Breathe. And begin.

Since I first picked up this book, where have I been?

What have I done?

Who have I met?

How have I felt in myself?

What challenges did I face along the way?

How am I feeling today?

NEVER CAN SAY GOODBYE

OK, we'll admit it. We hate goodbyes. And we're not going to let you go that easily. We would love to know if and how this book has helped you become a mindful drinker. We are committed to making Club Soda better for our members, and we want to know what worked and what didn't work. So please tell us what you think. We've created a special section of our website so you can tell us about your experiences:

joinclubsoda.com/how-to-be-a-mindful-drinker

AND FINALLY

Remember:

Always be brave, be honest, and be kind to yourself.
Live the life you imagine.
Become who you are.

What risks did I take?

What haven't I been able to do yet?

What have I learned about myself?

What has surprised me?

What's next?

What am I grateful for?

DRU IS PROUD TO BE PART
OF THE MINDFUL DRINKING MOVEMENT

HOW I CHANGED MY DRINKING: **DRU'S STORY**

The story of my drinking is so unremarkable, I've wondered if it's even worth telling. But then something happened that changed my mind.

I was out for dinner with friends, including someone I hadn't seen for a few years. I sat there with my alcohol-free cocktail and told her I was writing this book. We chatted about it and she was so supportive. I left feeling really good.

Afterward, I found out she'd messaged a mutual friend: "I didn't know Dru had a drinking problem?"

The truth is, I didn't. And that's not why I'm a mindful drinker.

When I was young, I never really got into the habit of getting drunk. I found a job straight out of school, got married, and had a child, so while other people my age were partying hard, my late nights were full of changing diapers.

Then, in my 30s, divorce happened. With some free weekends and a bit of money to spend, I made up for lost time! Sure, there were hangovers and nights I regret now, but there were lots of really good times, too. Some of those years are a bit of a blur, but I honestly thought that was just the trade-off everyone made.

In all that time, I never really thought about drinking at all. It was just something that happened, almost completely unconsciously. Looking back, I feel so lucky that I was always able to stop when I had to. If it wasn't for my son, I might have gone completely off the rails, and I'm so grateful for him.

When I met Laura, and we talked about her idea that became Club Soda, I thought it was just about helping other people. It seems so naive now, but I genuinely didn't realize it would help me change my drinking, too. But over time, I've discovered I prefer socializing when I'm not drunk. I deal with my anxiety better if I'm present to what's going on. And I've started getting really comfortable in my own skin. Bit by bit, I've put alcohol in its place.

And I've realized why I need to tell my unremarkable story. Because mindful drinking isn't just for people who have a "drinking problem" like my friend thought. It's also for people like me who never really think about drinking at all.

Maybe especially for people like me. If I know anything now, it's that anyone can be a mindful drinker.

MY STORY:
WHAT'S NEXT FOR ME?

THIS SPACE IS FOR YOUR LAST NOTES.
TAKE TIME TO REFLECT AND LOOK BACK
AT EVERYTHING THAT'S HAPPENED, AND
LOOK FORWARD TO YOUR FUTURE, TOO.

These notes pages work alongside the prompts across pages 212–213.
Complete in the spaces below or copy into your journal or notebook.

REFLECTION AND PLANNING

Since I first picked up this book, where have I been?

What have I done?

Who have I met?

How have I felt in myself?

How am I feeling today?

What challenges did I face along the way?

What risks did I take?

What has surprised me?

What have I learned about myself?

What haven't I been able to do yet?

What am I grateful for?

What's next?

INDEX

AUTHORS AND ACKNOWLEDGMENTS

Dru Jaeger is a writer and researcher who is passionate about the well-being of people and the planet.

Anja Madhvani is a drinks specialist and writer with an interest in cultural identity and behavior change.

Laura Willoughby is a community campaigner who believes that social movements can change anything, even our personal drinking habits.

Jussi Tolvi is a social scientist and statistician who is fascinated by the behavior of individuals and groups.

The authors are proud to work for Club Soda. We want to thank the rest of the team for everything they do.

We are who we are because of every Club Soda member. Thanks especially to Brynn, Butch, Jack, Melissa, and Sarah for your stories, and to Alison, Barbara, Cathy, Claire, Deborah, Donna, Emma, Glen, Hanban, Helen, Jacquie, Jen, Jimmy, Jo, Joanne, Judy, Julie, Karren, Laura, Liz, Martin, Mary, Melanie, Neil, Rachel, Rosie, Sandra, Sara, Sean, and Zoe.

So many people and organizations are involved in making a mindful drinking movement happen, it's impossible to mention everyone who has helped us over the years. Support from the Wellcome Trust, Bethnal Green Ventures, and Big Society Capital made writing this book possible. And special thanks are due to Amy and Fiona at Clever Together and Jo and Nick at OSCA for your insights into Club Soda members' intentions and stories of change.

We are profoundly grateful to Nikki, Amy, Stephanie, Mary-Clare, and everyone at DK. This book wouldn't have happened without you.

And finally, thanks to you for reading this book. If you ever meet us in real life, yes, we'd love a drink. Thanks for the offer. Let's see what this place has for mindful drinkers ...

PUBLISHER'S ACKNOWLEDGMENTS
The publisher would like to thank Lucy Philpott and Millie Andrew for editorial assistance and Hilary Bird for indexing.

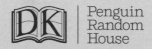

Senior Editor Nikki Sims
Editor Amy Slack
US Editor Megan Douglass
Art Editor Amy Child
Jacket Co-ordinator Lucy Philpott
Jacket Designer Amy Cox
Producer, Pre-production David Almond
Senior Producer Stephanie McConnell
Managing Editor Stephanie Farrow
Managing Art Editor Christine Keilty
Publisher Mary-Clare Jerram
Art Director Maxine Pedliham

First American Edition, 2019
Published in the United States by DK Publishing
1450 Broadway, Suite 801, New York, NY 10018

A catalog record for this book
is available from the Library of Congress.
ISBN 978-1-4654-9247-0

Printed and bound in Canada

A WORLD OF IDEAS:
SEE ALL THERE IS TO KNOW
www.dk.com